S. HRG. 103–999

ACCESS TO HEALTH CARE IN RURAL AND INNER CITY COMMUNITIES UNDER HEALTH CARE REFORM

HEARING

BEFORE THE

COMMITTEE ON FINANCE
UNITED STATES SENATE

ONE HUNDRED THIRD CONGRESS

SECOND SESSION

APRIL 21, 1994

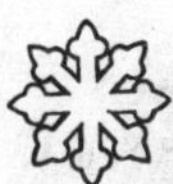

Printed for the use of the Committee on Finance

U.S. GOVERNMENT PRINTING OFFICE

WASHINGTON : 1994

85–462—CC

For sale by the U.S. Government Printing Office
Superintendent of Documents, Congressional Sales Office, Washington, DC 20402
ISBN 0-16-046892-2

(II)

CONTENTS

OPENING STATEMENT

COMMITTEE PRESS RELEASE

PUBLIC WITNESSES

ALPHABETICAL LISTING AND APPENDIX MATERIAL SUBMITTED

COMMUNICATIONS

ACCESS TO HEALTH CARE IN RURAL AND INNER CITY COMMUNITIES UNDER HEALTH CARE REFORM

THURSDAY, APRIL 21, 1994

U.S. SENATE,
COMMITTEE ON FINANCE,
Washington, DC.

The hearing was convened, pursuant to notice, at 10:00 a.m., in room SD–215, Dirksen Senate Office Building, Hon. Daniel Patrick Moynihan (chairman of the committee) presiding.

Also present: Senators Baucus, Pryor, Conrad, Packwood, Dole, Roth, Chafee, Durenberger, and Grassley.

[The press release announcing the hearing follows:]

[Press Release No. H–26, April 18, 1994]

FINANCE COMMITTEE SETS HEARING ON RURAL AND URBAN HEALTH CARE

WASHINGTON, DC—Senator Daniel Patrick Moynihan (D–NY), Chairman of the Senate Committee on Finance, announced today that the Committee will continue its examination of health care issues with a hearing on access to health care in rural and urban communities.

The hearing will begin at *10:00 A.M. on Thursday, April 21, 1994* in room SD–215 of the Dirksen Senate Office Building.

"Rural and inner city communities share many of the same problems—shortages of providers, high numbers of uninsured, and significant populations with poor health status," Senator Moynihan said in announcing the hearing. "The Committee will examine how proposed health care reforms would affect the medical and related services delivered in these communities."

OPENING STATEMENT OF HON. DANIEL PATRICK MOYNIHAN, A U.S. SENATOR FROM NEW YORK, CHAIRMAN, COMMITTEE ON FINANCE

The CHAIRMAN. A very good morning. My goodness, are we not all alert and on hand. This is the most recent and one of the concluding hearings of the Committee on Finance on health care matters. Our subject today is access to health services in rural and inner city communities under various health care reform proposals.

We will be to some extent. I think, discussing inner cities first and rural areas second.

We welcome our distinguished panelists and our guests. First, Dr. Mark Smith, who is executive vice president of the Kaiser Family Foundation from Menlo Park, CA. Dr. Smith, we welcome you.

We would like to ask our witnesses, as we have a double panel, to keep within their appointed time, but not too severely. I think if you have concluding thoughts, by all means let us hear them.

Good morning, Dr. Smith.

STATEMENT OF MARK D. SMITH, M.D., EXECUTIVE VICE PRESIDENT, HENRY J. KAISER FAMILY FOUNDATION, MENLO PARK, CA

Dr. SMITH. Good morning, Senator. Thank you very much for the invitation. We are here to talk about access to care for urban and rural populations. I have expanded my thoughts a little bit to include other people who are underserved.

You have with you today as other witnesses people who work on the front lines in a number of the institutions that care for these populations and I will not attempt to speak directly to their conditions or their institution's needs. But I would like to briefly take up with you several conceptual points that I think are important as you consider health care reform in terms of how it affects these populations.

I should start by telling you that I am both a physician—most of my work has been with AIDS for the last 8 to 10 years—and an MBA. I suppose that makes me among the more detested and despised people, depending on your point of view in this system. But it does seem to me that it is useful to combine both the compassion and caring for which physicians are trained and some practical sense of what the bottom line is and that is what your committee's very difficult balance in that——

The CHAIRMAN. That has been a tension we have had for the whole year.

Dr. SMITH. Yes, me, too.

I want to make essentially five points. The first is that the health care system is changing dramatically, independently of what this committee or the Congress does. And it is important when thinking about trying to solve the problems of underserved populations to solve the problems of the system as it is now and as it is becoming and not the system as it was 10 to 15 years ago.

In particular, that means the system is becoming more organized, more aggregated, more integrated, more corporatized. I happen to welcome that on many fronts, but I recognize that it does pose some problems and it is the special problems of vulnerable populations in such a system and not in the old cottage industry fee-for-service industry that I believe this committee must address.

I think that means that new models of managed care are necessary, since managed care is here to stay, and you will hear about some exciting new models today. Those models must be developed and supported. They also must be evaluated because the incentive system in American medicine is now changing from one in which one gets more if one does more to one in which one gets more if one does less.

Both incentive systems have potential for abuses, but I believe that poor people and older people and isolated people and sick people are perhaps particularly vulnerable under the latter system; and, therefore, there is also a need for the development of objective standards of quality of care. This is a development that is already going on quite a bit in private industry.

But I believe that in a number of areas such as substance abuse, mental health, care of complex diseases like HIV, there may not be sufficient incentive in the private sector to develop measures of standards of quality so as to assure ourselves and ensure the public that people are receiving high quality care.

The third point has to do with so-called enabling services. I direct you, if I may, to Figure 3 in my prepared testimony, which was a very modest study performed for our foundation by Dr. Tracy Lieu, looking at people who use public immunization clinics and Contra Costa County, California in the fall of 1992.

The interesting result of the study is that a majority of the people using public immunization clinics in Contra Costa County had health insurance. Some had MediCal, a majority, about 22 percent; 34 percent had private health insurance.

First of all, many of them did not know that they had coverage for immunizations. But even people who had insurance cited other problems with their insurance as the reason that they were attending public clinics—sometimes transportation, sometimes waiting times, sometimes language.

The public sector has filled an important gap for people who do not have health insurance in this country. And it seems to me that particularly when some services such as transportation, and to a lesser extent translation, are currently reimbursed under Medicaid, that how one pays for these important enablers of use of the medical care system, particularly for people who have severe disabilities, is going to be an important thing to consider.

The fourth point has to do with legal protections. There is, as you certainly know better than I, an enormous amount of money at stake in this system. I believe that most managed care administrators, physicians, and operators are honest, capable, professional, and want to do the best for their patients and enrollees, but we are all aware of some abuses.

Independent of bad will, the sheer creation of bureaucracy of the kinds of size of plans that are now being developed means that there will be inertia and red tape. So I believe that legal protections are necessary.

The last point is the one that I would like to leave you with, particularly, and that has to do with the matter of risk adjustment or premium adjustment. Let me give you an example from someone with AIDS.

If I had AIDS and have a condition called CMV retinitis, a sight-threatening condition, under the kind of underwriting reform your committee is now contemplating, reforms which I support—the elimination of pre-existing condition, community rating, et cetera—I would be allowed to walk into my local health insurer and demand that he or she write me a policy and demand that that policy be at the community rate, say $180 a month, despite the fact that my condition will cost more like $180 an hour, at least for the next several weeks.

So in my last chart I showed you some pretty good numbers which are there for ball parks of what the standard premium is and what the cost of AIDS care is. I believe that this committee must grapple with the question of some sort of spreading of the risk, lest the insurers, even those who are prohibited by law from refusing individuals, do everything in their power to market to the healthy and de-market the sick.

Thank you very much.

4

[The prepared statement of Dr. Smith appears in the appendix.]

The CHAIRMAN. Thank you, Dr. Smith.

We will have questions at the end. Now, we are going to hear next from Dr. Stanley Block, who is Medical Director of the Ambulatory Health Care Foundation, Inc., at Providence, RI. And providentially, the Senator from Rhode Island is here to introduce Dr. Block.

Senator CHAFEE. Well, Mr. Chairman, it is with great——

The CHAIRMAN. I thought that went very nicely—providentially. Do not act like you did not hear it. [Laughter.]

Senator CHAFEE. Mr. Chairman, I just want to say that it is so appropriate that we have testifying today on a panel dealing with the inner city service for health care Dr. Stanley Block.

Every single one of us on this committee are strongly in favor of community health centers. We all say that and we believe in it. But Dr. Stanley Block is someone who is right out in the trenches. I have been to his clinic. I have seen it in the late afternoon and early evenings just alive with patients who have come in there; and it shows what these community health care centers can do.

In our State they are very, very important. One-third of all our Medicaid patients are served by community health centers. In other words, that is where they get their medical health care.

When we talk community health centers, you are not just talking providing health services, you are talking overcoming language barriers. You are talking nutrition advice. You are talking what you might call holistic medicine.

In addition to that, it is a one-stop shopping place where they can get help with housing and clothing. I have been to one of his centers, his very center where they had a rack where those who chose to contribute clothes would contribute them and indigent families could obtain some additional clothing.

So you could not have chosen a better witness than Dr. Stanley Block. It is with great pride that I introduce him to this committee.

The CHAIRMAN. We thank you, Senator Chafee.

Good morning, Dr. Block.

STATEMENT OF STANLEY H. BLOCK, M.D., MEDICAL DIRECTOR, AMBULATORY HEALTH CARE FOUNDATION, INC., PROVIDENCE, RI

Dr. BLOCK. Well, thank you so much, gentlemen, for the kind opportunity to testify before you today. I have had the pleasure of serving as a medical director and pediatrician at the Providence Ambulatory Health Care Foundation for 17 years now. We serve about 24,000 patients who make about 70,000 visits to our doctors and our nurse practitioners each year.

Almost all of our patients are poor or near poor. We receive a Federal grant under Section 330 of the Public Health Service Act, so that we have never had to turn away a single patient for primary care in the last quarter center because of inability to pay.

Across the nation there are 700 centers like ours and they serve about 7 million Americans in need. In my opinion, the community health centers have been one of the greatest successes in the health care industry that this Nation is seeing. A small investment of Federal dollars has given an enormous bang for the buck for those in need.

As someone who spent a couple of decades in the inner city, I feel that the enactment of the essential community provider integration clause, like that agreed unanimously by the House Ways and Means Health Subcommittee last month, which would require health plans to contract with FQHCs (Federally Qualified Health Centers) and pay us adequately to cover the inherent higher costs of treating the underserved, is critical.

Why do we need health centers after health care reform? Even if every American is provided a ticket to health care, health centers, I feel, need to be fully included and expanded to look after the needs of inner city and minority America.

Over the last several years, I have seen some tragedies when traditional health center patients have tried to access HMOs that are geared more to the middle class patients. HMOs and other mainstream providers have traditionally shunned the very patients that we have served. No wonder. It is certainly not that they are evil or bad.

But in looking at the bottom line, the patients that we serve in the inner city are the very highest risk patients. They have more of virtually every disease—more lead poisoning, TB, blood pressure problems, AIDS, substance abuse. I can go on and on. They have language barriers, cultural barriers, many are non-compliant.

And certainly this is the very worst selection that an HMO could make if they are worried about the bottom line. Health centers on the other hand have cared for these populations for a quarter of a century.

From our State's HMONG population we heard about the father of a little HMONG baby who had received HMO coverage through his factory job and the dad called the HMO that he had joined and told the doctors in the few words of English that he knew, "Baby sick, baby very sick."

And the doctor—who is actually an acquaintance of mine, an excellent pediatrician—tried to find out what was wrong. The father could only say in a few broken words of English, "chicken pox," and the pediatrician told him that they would see him on Monday when the HMO opened.

Now the pediatrician apparently did not know that when a HMONG father calls up about a child's illness something is usually dreadfully wrong. Nor could the pediatrician understand that HMONG parents and Southeast Asian parents in general usually do not show the terror that a middle class family would show if their baby was dying.

Sadly, the little HMONG baby did die of overwhelming infection before Monday's appointment.

The CHAIRMAN. Was it chicken pox?

Dr. BLOCK. From what I understand, it was a bacterial infection that was a super infection above and beyond the chicken pox.

The CHAIRMAN. He had symptoms of.

Dr. BLOCK. Right.

And this is one of the very best HMOs. Now if this can happen in one of the nation's premier HMOs, you can only imagine what can happen in those that are less interested in patients' welfare and care.

I saw another Hispanic baby whose mom confused Ipecac with an antibiotic, both of which were prescribed in an excellent local hospital. The mom was giving the Ipecac three times a day which could have killed the baby, and kept the antibiotic on the shelf to be used in case of poisoning, the very opposite of what the physician had meant.

That was because nobody could explain in terms that she could understand that the antibiotic was for the infection and the Ipecac was in case in the future the child ever were poisoned, which is standard of care for health maintenance in children. We try to prevent tragedies like this from occurring by having translators on site.

I also wonder whether traditional providers in HMOs and other health care facilities are going to address the wrong phone numbers and the wrong addresses that patients give us. I cared for a baby whose blood culture grew out at 48 hours meningococcemia, which is a dreadful bacteria that kills fairly quickly.

The mom had given us the wrong address and the wrong phone number and we had no way of contacting her to alert her that her baby had this terrible infection. Now whether she was an undocumented alien or for whatever reasons, she gave us incorrect information. The police could not find her. Through a community network and working with the police, we eventually tracked her down. But will HMOs be willing to invest the time and effort needed to protect these babies lives? I should add that this baby did very well in the hospital getting the appropriate antibiotics.

I do not think that these instances will show up in quality measures or consumer report cards because, though they are tragic, they are relatively infrequent. Therefore, it is critical that this committee protect such patients and such communities.

Representatives John Lewis and Fred Grandy, the authors of the Ways and Means provision, have said this far more eloquently than I could say it.

The CHAIRMAN. Why do you not tell us what they said?

Dr. BLOCK. Essentially what they are saying is, that they feel it is a requirement that health plans doing business in the underserved inner city and rural communities contract with essential community providers serving those areas and pay them adequately.

They go on to explain all of the reasons they believe that requiring health plans to contract with essential providers in underserved areas is the most appropriate way to ensure an equitable sharing of responsibility for care of high risk populations and to safeguard this vital, yet fragile infrastructure.

In Rhode Island, through a Social Security Act Section 1115 waiver, Medicaid patients are now being required to join HMOs. We are concerned that this entire program is underfunded and that care will be sporadic and that patients will suffer.

One of the major HMOs had offered to contract with us at half of the cost base reimbursement that we presently get. This could erode the financial viability of community health centers. And, frankly, I doubt if the HMOs, once the health centers fade away from the scene, will be willing to take on the duties that the health centers have taken on for a quarter of a century.

I should also add that since Medicaid patients go on and off of Medicaid rolls, I doubt that HMOs will see the long-term savings from the initial preventive care that they give, which after all is a basic premise of most managed care programs.

In other words, if you put in initial dollars to preventive care in a managed care environment, one expects to be able to reap the benefits of a healthy patient and a lower cost of care later on. But if the patients in a Medicaid program are going on and off the Medicaid rolls, as they do in Rhode Island and I am sure in other parts of the country, I do not think that those savings will be realized by the managed care industry.

Because of the high risk nature of patients that we see and the fact that over half of our patients speak no English and have no phone, the cost of managing their care is certainly going to be higher than that of a suburban family. How do you manage the care of a patient and get prior approval for an emergency room visit if the patient cannot call you or speak your language?

Will HMOs and other traditional providers be willing to educate the inner city and minority patients as the health centers have done? We just saw a 6-week-old baby who stopped breathing and had what we considered a near miss SIDS, or Sudden Infant Death Syndrome.

Now we got the baby an apnea alarm, and taught the mother through a Cambodian interpreter how to give CPR should this occur again. The mother came back a week later and was very proud and said, "I saved the baby's life (through a Cambodian interpreter) five times when the baby stopped breathing and turned desperately blue."

We said, "Well, why did you not take the baby to the hospital and call 911 and get there right away?" She said, "I did not know I had to."

Now this gives you some idea of the lack of sophistication of many of the patients we see and the enormous amount of effort that goes into trying to teach patients how to care for sick children.

Now I know that there is no less popular topic in health care reform than the provision of care to illegal immigrants. I think American taxpayers can rightfully ask whether it is their obligation to pay for medical care for those who enter our Nation illegally. But self-interest, I would think, should dictate that all of us have some stake in the basic health care of even illegal immigrants since our own children are going to be exposed to drug resistant tuberculosis and other diseases from undeveloped countries.

And unless our border policies change, which is way beyond the scope of my expertise——

The CHAIRMAN. Of this hearing.

Dr. BLOCK. The immigrants who come in illegally and with no documentation are going to continue to enter our inner cities and rural areas. I think it is in everyone's interest that they receive proper immunizations, tuberculosis treatment and other care to prevent America's public health from being jeopardized.

One-third of our pregnant women are undocumented. Of course, most of our patients are working poor and near poor people. But about one-third of our pregnant women are undocumented aliens. I wonder whether traditional HMOs would want to care for them even after health care reform.

The CHAIRMAN. That, of course, we will get to. Dr. Block, we thank you very, very much. We have had a hearing on this subject and it is difficult to legislate for persons who are technically in violation of statute. It is one of those complexities.

Dr. Delgado, who is president and chief executive officer of the National Coalition of Hispanic Health and Human Services Organizations. Dr. Delgado, we welcome you.

STATEMENT OF JANE L. DELGADO, PH. D., PRESIDENT AND CHIEF EXECUTIVE OFFICER, NATIONAL COALITION OF HISPANIC HEALTH AND HUMAN SERVICES ORGANIZATIONS, WASHINGTON, DC

Dr. DELGADO. I am glad to be here. I am here representing an organization that is 21 years old and has 350 organizational members and 1,000 individuals who provide front line health and human services to Hispanic communities.

Thirty-nine percent of our people are uninsured and most of them, 82 percent, are uninsured because they work in jobs that do not provide any health care. They are the working poor who have no health care.

Additionally, our members are people who spent days wrestling with some of the hard issues because so much of health care reform affects us. We convened a meeting of 68 of our leaders around the country. As you can imagine, it was quite an interesting meeting since we kept everyone together in a room to debate and come up with our solutions, which were in three areas.

One was reducing the bureaucracy. Two was increasing revenue and costs. And three, to ensure quality. In reducing the bureaucracy, one of the key things we always talk about is that we believe in true universal coverage and we say very strongly that not covering undocumented persons is an administrative and bureaucratic nightmare.

When you ask a firefighter to put out a fire, you do not ask him to check on the legal status of the people in the building. You just tell him to put out the fire. There are health fires in our communities. Up until now, every public health law has been silent on the issue of legal status. To change that is regressive. If you look at every nation that has national health insurance, they cover everyone. I, myself, have my own Japanese health insurance card, having had the misfortune of being sick there.

One of the things we keep emphasizing is coverage of all residents is in the public health interest. An example is with HIV. Immigrants to this country have a very low rate of HIV. However, after being here, their rates seem to go up. So it is not just that people come here with illness, but once here they get exposed to a whole host of health risks. Furthermore, data from the Department of Justice shows that in the prior year to legalization only 4 percent of the people who were legalized and had hospital visits, had those hospital visits paid for in free care.

It may be good politics not to include undocumented persons, but it is bad medicine. It is bad health.

We also are concerned about Puerto Rico. People say, well, Puerto Rico is different. But Puerto Ricans are Americans. They are U.S. citizens. And they will not be getting the same level of care as other people. This not only affects Puerto Rico but all the States where Puerto Ricans live. Because as we well know, there is a very strong tie between the island and the mainland.

The other thing which we are concerned about in reducing the bureaucracy is the need to include a full package of mental health benefits. Many people are not talking about this. But for Hispanics who have the highest rate of attempted suicides among adolescents and for our people who have very high rates of depression, we are very concerned about having good mental health benefits and not something that is phased in over time.

But we are also a responsible group. So when we talked about comprehensive and universal coverage we also talked about raising revenue. We talked about taxes on tobacco, alcohol and guns. And among those 68 people, I can tell you, our hunters from Texas were not too thrilled about that gun tax. But as a community, all these people decided that we would support this.

I do not have to tell you about the importance of taxing tobacco, especially in our community where we are targeted by the tobacco industry to increase our level of smoking. The number of Hispanics in the United States, is 1½ times the number of Australians in Australia. So if you are talking about markets, that is a very large market.

Think of how the tobacco industry sees us. They do not see us as a minority, they see us as a very large market. And unfortunately, our youth and our women are suffering from that.

The last area is the area of ensuring quality through cultural and linguistically competent systems. And people ask, Jane, what on earth do you mean by that. Does everyone have to speak Spanish? Does everyone have to understand that, you know, being Hispanic is more than having Taco Tuesday in the cafeteria?

The answer is, people have to be able to understand another person's culture. Part of that is best shown in a study that appeared in the Journal of the American Medical Association in March of 1993 that looked at Hispanics who went into the UCLA Emergency Room. When they controlled for gender, language ability and insurance status, the best predictor of whether or not someone got a pain killer if someone had a broken leg is whether or not they were Hispanic.

Obviously, access is an issue. But we have to ensure that equality of access also means equality of outcome. I think too often we loose sight of that.

Finally, the whole issue of infrastructure. Yes, community health centers are critical. But you cannot put all of the responsibility on them. There are too few of them and too few of them serving any of the low income communities.

You know, the community health centers only serve 13 percent of the eligible populations in poverty. You cannot put it all on them. You have to extend that to other kinds of providers in the communities. For Hispanics this is even more important because so many of our providers are not federally qualified community health centers. This is a difficult time for us and we want to make sure that we have good data so we understand where people receive services.

Along these lines the final thing to remember is that in your quest to have good access you need good outcome data. Current plans talk about having a universal health claim form but do not have a race/ethnic identifier.

Current data shows that the black community does not live very long. Hispanics have a health profile similar to women; we live a long time, but we have a lot of chronic illness. When you clump us together as a minority, the black community looks healthier and we sort of look healthy because people assumed that we did not live a long time. This is incorrect. Equality of access is important. Make sure you make certain that whatever you do has equality of outcome, too.

Thank you.

The CHAIRMAN. Thank you, Dr. Delgado.

[The prepared statement of Dr. Delgado appears in the appendix.]

The CHAIRMAN. We are addressing that claim form matter without any very great expectation of success.

Now we are going to hear from Eugene McCabe, who is the Director of the North General Hospital in New York City at 122nd and Madison Avenue. It is now, since you have finished your work, a 240-bed teaching hospital. Something in that range. We welcome you, Mr. McCabe.

STATEMENT OF EUGENE L. McCABE, PRESIDENT AND CHIEF EXECUTIVE OFFICER, NORTH GENERAL HOSPITAL, NEW YORK, NY

Mr. McCABE. Thank you, Mr. Chairman. I would like to acknowledge the work you have done on behalf of North General Hospital and other hospitals in New York City as well.

North General has a long history of service to Harlem and has developed the unique understanding of the health care issues endemic to a largely Medicaid uninsured and underinsured patient population. I appreciate the opportunity to help identify the elements I believe must be considered in the design of standards for improved access to care and to assist in defining the provisions for quality services that would be a part of a reformed health care landscape.

As we view the progress of health care reform, it appears certain that the final bill will be constructed from a variety of principles shared by the administration, the Senate and the House. But no matter what the origin, we believe universal access is key to any reform package.

We also strongly believe that the essential community provider provision in the administration bill should be strengthened to reflect the role physicians and hospitals serving areas like Harlem have played historically and continue to play despite many obstacles.

Each day the media reports the inexorable movement towards the creation of networks by health care providers to merger, acquisition or affiliation. The underlying reasons for this consolidation—which by the way we agree with—are projected to reduce costs and improve services.

If, indeed, this is to be the new world of health care, providers in the Harlems across the country share basic concerns. Will their current role be compromised? Will they have the opportunity to participate in these networks? Will their unique relationship with their patients change?

Last Thursday in a meeting with Harlem physicians at North General, First Lady Hillary Rodham Clinton heard firsthand the concerns of minority providers regarding reform. The consensus at that meeting was that it would inexcusable if a consequence of seeking to improve health care in Harlem was to lock out providers that have rendered quality service to this population for so long.

These concerns are expressed throughout New York City as well. As Senator Moynihan well knows, it is a fact that our city shoulders a larger burden of the nation's health care ills. For example, 1.5 million New Yorkers lack insurance coverage. While the city's Medicaid and uncompensated care expenditures continue to grow expedentially, there has been nonmeasurable improvement in health status and it could get worse.

Frankly stated, some compute models suggest a significant impact on New York City hospitals under current estimates. Specifically, it has been projected that some reform measures could result in a $30 million loss for North General. If extrapolated over the vista of New York City hospitals, we are talking about billions of dollars being drained from an already unstable system.

However, we clearly support the need for reform because each day we witness the ravages of a system where many are denied prompt and effective care. Our overused emergency room and under utilized primary care services drive up costs, creating instability in an already overburdened system.

Every day we see patients who only seek care when a chronic problem is escalated to an acute level. When this happens, care is often less effective and always more expensive. Last year at North General we provided 25,000 emergency room visits. The majority of these were to patients in need of basic primary care.

Moreover, the 100,000 ambulatory care visits we provide at the hospital each year could be better served by managed care in less expensive settings. Despite these dyer possibilities, we welcome change and believe the time for reform is now.

We view this as an opportunity for North General and community physicians to participate in shaping the future of health care delivery in our neighborhoods. In anticipation of change, we have implemented programs to link patients with primary care providers. We educate our patients about preventive care and how to access the system.

Though we have done a lot of work in this area, much more remains to be done. Our patients' priorities are often something other than prevention. Any new delivery system has to consider the episodic manner in which they access care and its impact on their health and health care expenditures.

We played a leading role in the development of a service delivery network organized to increase access, ensure quality and promote cost efficiencies. The network will integrate the service of hospital and physicians, a home health care agency, a long term care facility and ambulatory care satellites.

By forming this network, this group of providers will assume fiscal and clinical responsibility for the provision of high quality services to our patients. Thus, we are currently a step ahead of the game. We operate a sophisticated management information system that will drive the network, share data and facilitate access to patient information.

Based on our service and the Federal designation of our service grid as a health manpower shortage area, our network meets all the qualifications of an essential community provider. What concerns us, however, is the level of support in the bill that will be provided to ECPs.

Limited grant awards have been offered in various proposals, which based on our experience will fall far short of the expenses associated with network building. Protected costs for primary care site development, MIS, planning, staff recruitment, training and health promotion will exceed proposed subsidies in an area where strategic investment can significantly reduce costs.

Moreover, funding for enabling services such as outreach and social services, both required by grants supported ECPs, should not be addressed through a separate mechanism. Instead, these activities should be financed through development grants.

We believe that larger, better financed health plans that do not qualify for ECP funding must also be required to offer enabling services if they choose to target this population. This revision to the bill will level the playing field.

Hospitals and physicians that have served populations like ours have had limited access to capital for plant, equipment and MIS infrastructure. Grant funds and loans must be sufficient to support the development of those systems so that we can effectively compete with the large private health plans who will find our patients attractive once they have access to a health security card.

Additional access points for primary care services will be required if we are serious about redirecting health utilization patterns. For providers in urban areas, tax incentives for capital formation are vital for expansion. This will be money well spent when you consider the savings associated with keeping people out of emergency rooms and costly inpatient settings.

In closing, the health care market is already moving towards reform. North General and other health care facilities have dealt with issues of access, quality care, and cost containment in low income communities long before reform became part of the public debate. We have weathered inadequate reimbursement methodologies, high costs from serving sicker patients that use hospitals for emergencies and difficulty in retaining qualified physicians.

We believe that improving these conditions is possible if reform recognizes that those who have been doing the job need new tools to compete in the new environment.

Thank you very much.

The CHAIRMAN. We thank you, sir. I ought to note that you were a member of Governor Cuomo's Task Force to Review the Clinton Administration's Health Care Reform Plan. So I assume from your statement that it has been projected that some reform measures could result in a $30 million loss for North General, specifically you are talking about the Clinton plan.

Mr. McCABE. Yes, we are.

The CHAIRMAN. Thank you very much.

[The prepared statement of Mr. McCabe appears in the appendix.]

The CHAIRMAN. And now to make the case for HMOs, Dr. Clyde Oden, Jr., who is president and CEO of Watts Health Foundation of Inglewood, CA. Good morning, Dr. Oden. Thank you for coming all this way.

STATEMENT OF DR. CLYDE W. ODEN, JR., M.D., PRESIDENT AND CHIEF EXECUTIVE OFFICER, WATTS HEALTH FOUNDATION, INC., INGLEWOOD, CA

Dr. ODEN. Good morning, Mr. Chairman. Thank you so very much for the opportunity to testify before this committee.

I am the Rev. Dr. Clyde W. Oden, Jr. president and chief executive officer of the Watts Health Foundation and its HMO, the United Health Plan. My complete testimony has been presented to you in writing.

The CHAIRMAN. It will be placed in the record.

[The prepared statement of Dr. Oden appears in the appendix.]

Dr. ODEN. I would like, however, just to make several points.

The CHAIRMAN. You came all the way from California. Make all the points you want. [Laughter.]

Dr. ODEN. Well, thank you. Then let me take off my coat. [Laughter.]

First of all, my sense of history, compassion and patriotism says that this Congress should not adjourn without there being meaningful health reform passed for the citizens of this country. That this opportunity should not be missed. That irrespective of ideology and particular positions, the American people need to be assured that regardless of where they work, whether it is a large company or a small company, no matter where they live, whether it is a rural area or an urban area, no matter what language is spoken at home, no matter what their race or creed, they should have the assurance that they have health care coverage as a right and not as a privilege.

Beyond that, there are some points I would like to make in terms of our specific experience, in terms of providing care to urban and inner city areas. Our organization has had 27 years of experience, both by working as a community health center, which is where we started, as the Watts Health Center, and as an HMO where we have served low-income communities for 21 years.

And having both the experiences of serving as a community health center, which we still do, and serving populations under managed care, we are convinced that managed care is the best alternative available for these populations given certain conditions and circumstances that I think are important and are indicated in my written testimony.

Beyond that, it is important to understand that in order to improve the tragic health statistics that we find in many of our urban centers it is necessary to go beyond just paying for health care. It goes beyond just seeing that there are providers in communities. There has to be active promotion of both appropriate life style behavior and promotion of preventive and primary health care.

Community health centers have been and are a very excellent alternative and delivery point for providing care in inner city areas. I believe that community health centers ought to be promoted and that there ought to be more of them throughout the United States.

But beyond that, there needs to be resources made available to community health centers that will allow them to more actively participate in the managed care environment, and that means investment with respect to infrastructure development, investment for systems and technology development, investments for training and retraining of staff and Boards, and capital in order to allow them to better assume risk.

But I would also say that in terms of serving inner city and urban areas, with respect to managed care, mandating any group providers to participate does something about the issue of accountability. If on one hand we are going to hold systems accountable, and they should be held publicly accountable, if they are going to have to report how well they perform, then they have to be able to hold every provider in their system accountable.

And if there are any entitled providers who do not really have to respond to the necessities of this kind of accountability, I think we create more problems than we solve in terms of solutions to this issue.

Second, with respect to providing cost effective care, premium regulations and price caps work less well than competition for informed consumers. We are seeing the experience currently in California where the costs of care is moderating significantly because there is open and appropriate competition for patients who are looking for high quality, low-cost care that is both culturally appropriate for them, as well as satisfying them in terms of the services that are provided.

Essentially, community providers must be allowed to participate in health reform. But they need to be empowered through investments so that they can participate, rather than necessarily mandated in order to participate without giving them infrastructure development. That is just so very important.

Finally, the principles of universal coverage, local accessibility to primary and preventive care, insurance reform so that persons are not denied coverage with regard to their health status or previous health status, choice of providers and managed competition are the most appropriate features in any health care reform.

Thank you so very much.

The CHAIRMAN. Thank you, Dr. Oden.

Well, we have heard a range of views stated with moderation, which we appreciate. If I heard one thing this morning, all of you are telling us that we should not set about to reform a health care system that no longer exists.

I see you nodding. All right, we have to make the point that the reporter cannot record a nod.

Dr. SMITH. I agree, sir.

The CHAIRMAN. You said there was a time, if I recall correctly, that if you did more you got more in the way of providing services. Now if you do more you might get less. This is changing from a demand system to a supply system.

Dr. SMITH. Right.

The CHAIRMAN. And you are picking up the same phenomenon in your research. I simply make the point, which Senator Dole might want to hear, Dr. Oden said that price caps will not do it, managed care will.

Senator DOLE. I read that.

The CHAIRMAN. You read that, did you? But here we are and good morning all. Now, Senator Dole, would you like to exercise the Leader's privilege of opening the questions?

Senator DOLE. Since I am late, I think I will wait and see what develops here.

The CHAIRMAN. Sure. Well, I think we simply have heard two sets of propositions. One is that the health care system has been changing rapidly and is becoming price sensitive in a way it has not been. The structures we have put in place were not price sensitive. For example, Medicaid is not price sensitive.

Could I just ask the panel if that is a feeling they have, that we have moved to a climate which is price sensitive?

Dr. SMITH. I think that is right. I think that is one of the positive features of managed care. As I said in my written testimony, a report from the Congressional Budget Office points out as it was attempting to measure the cost savings for managed care, it points out it is becoming increasingly hard because increasingly there is no alternative. Everything is managed care.

The old fee-for-service indemnity system in many places, such as California, no longer exists. And although there is considerable heterogeneity, that is certainly the direction that the country is moving.

The CHAIRMAN. Yes. We had a Dr. Schultze, who is a center colleague of yours, Dr. Oden. He runs the University of California Los Angeles Hospital. He was sitting there. That is the California seat.

Dr. ODEN. The California seat, yes.

The CHAIRMAN. This time last week he said, there is just no indemnity insurance left in Southern California. He said, we get some because there are people who traveled to the hospitals for special procedures, but otherwise that is something that has gone by.

Comments, Ms. Delgado?

Dr. DELGADO. Yes. I get very concerned when people focus on the whole issue of price sensitivity, assuming that that is good. You can be price sensitive, but unless you are measuring your outcomes, you are not going to know whether or not what you do is good.

The CHAIRMAN. We have heard that, too.

Dr. DELGADO. Yes. And that is a major concern.

The CHAIRMAN. We have heard very responsible people say we are going to get better and better, and then we might start getting less health care further into this continuum of being price sensitive.

We have heard academic health centers say, we are not efficient. No one wants to send anyone to our hospitals because we charge more because we teach doctors and nurses how to become doctors and nurses.

Mr. McCabe, you had something?

Mr. MCCABE. I think there are several phenomenon taking place in New York with regard to costs. I think on the one hand private for-profit managed care companies are coming in and making deals with hospitals. In some way the deal that they are trying to make now is about the same as it would cost to take care of patients in the way we do. But the feeling is that in order to get market share, they have to make a better deal at the front end.

The CHAIRMAN. Just listen to your language. In order to get market share.

Mr. MCCABE. Right.

The CHAIRMAN. That is how people who sell concrete talk.

Mr. MCCABE. Exactly. And I think one of the difficulties will be that when they do get this market share, then I think they are going to try to rachet down costs. The impact among hospitals is going to be significant.

I personally believe that hospital costs are too high. I think that you cannot afford to provide the care we do in New York under the system that we have now, and so we are going to have to have a transition. The issue would be, what happens during that transition and who will survive and who will not survive.

I think the issue in places like Harlem is even more difficult because you do have an experiment going on in Brooklyn, New York where you are signing up people for Medicaid managed care. The issue is that people are signing up and they are going in managed care programs and then they are getting off those programs. And in 70 percent of the cases these are the same people who present themselves at the emergency rooms in those hospitals.

So I think the issue has to be that it is going to be price sensitive. But what we are saying, and I think you heard from the panel, is that if you are going to have the essential community provider concept then you should give hospitals and doctors who are in those neighborhoods some ability to access capital so they can create these networks and I think over time change utilization and be able to do a better job at lesser costs.

The CHAIRMAN. A very good point.

Dr. Oden, you wanted to comment?

Dr. ODEN. Yes. I just wanted to say that what we are seeing fundamentally is a change to a buyer's market. And buyers are beginning to dictate whether that is the government acting as a more prudent purchaser or corporations or voluntary alliances. That is making all the providers and systems become more disciplined.

That is, in fact, affecting how costs are being passed through the system. I think it is important and that it is a major paradigm shift that we are seeing.

The CHAIRMAN. A major paradigm shift. I guess I would leave it with my comment simply that we do not want to write legislation designed to fix up problems in a system that previously existed. We want to address the one that is coming into being, for which I thank you all very much.

Senator Packwood?

Senator PACKWOOD. Mr. Chairman, I am always fascinated when very competent people doing roughly the same thing or access to the same information come down on opposite sides of an issue. Bob Dole, remember, was the only one here at the time, the extraordinary debate that we had on the anti-ballistic missile system when Stewart Symington and Scoop Jackson were two and three on the Armed Services Committee and we were 180 degrees opposite based upon the same facts.

I want to address this to Dr. Block and Dr. Oden. Dr. Block, I am reading from your testimony. "Many of the major proposals for health care reform, particularly the 'managed competition' approach which has received so much attention contained a lot of elements that raised concerns and whatnot." Then you just basically say, "managed competition will not do it."

Dr. Oden, who I think treats sort of the same kind of population says, "Our 21 years of experience operating a managed care system and our 27 years of being a fee-for—service provider have convinced that in the urban inner city context managed care is the superior accountable medical delivery system."

What is it that causes the two of you to come down almost opposite, I think serving roughly the same kinds of populations?

Dr. BLOCK. I do not know how many non-English speaking patients Dr. Oden's has had.

Dr. ODEN. There are 17 different languages that are spoken amongst the patients that we serve. In Los Angeles in particular, languages other than English are spoken quite frequently. We see a whole mixture of patients from different backgrounds and circumstances.

My position comes from experience—21 years experience—both trial and error. It has not always been easy.

Senator PACKWOOD. What I am intrigued with, I think Dr. Block comes from this long line of experience also and reaches an absolutely opposite conclusion.

Dr. DELGADO. But I think these gentlemen are no different than the members of the Senate who get facts and also come to different conclusions, too.

Senator PACKWOOD. They are not. [Laughter.]

What I am trying to find out is why they have come to a different conclusion.

Dr. BLOCK. Dr. Oden's HMO may be a very special and very excellent HMO. I am not convinced that at least in my experience I have seen HMOs in our area try to target the inner city, high risk low resource patient that requires an enormous amount of investment in time and money. It is bad for the bottom line.

They have traditionally avoided it, not because they are bad people or bad corporations, but because frankly they felt that they would go bankrupt doing it. Under the Medicaid managed care waiver in Rhode Island approved recently under an 1115 waiver, most of the HMOs have elected not to participate.

One of the reasons is that most of the HMOs that were asked and begged to participate on behalf of the State of Rhode Island feel that at least for the capitation rate that is offered with the resources that are available, this population is such a resource user, and the difficulty of managing care of people with no phones and no English is so difficult and costly, that they did not want to participate.

The tradition has been, for the 25 years that health centers have been in existence, that most HMOs—and I cannot speak for Dr. Oden's—but the vast majority of HMOs have shied away from the very inner city high risk areas that we are talking about.

Senator PACKWOOD. Dr. Oden?

Dr. ODEN. Senator Packwood, Los Angeles and Southern California is a far more mature market. We have had experience. We, not only our organization but many other managed care organizations, have had experiences serving underserved populations and now understand the situation better.

With respect to Medicaid in particular, our organization is partnering with seven other—six other for-profit and one other nonprofit—HMOs that serve Medicaid populations in Los Angeles County to bid together to serve that population.

Now that also is a change. But it is a change because we have been able to demonstrate that the mythology that it is too difficult and too expensive to serve low income populations is just that, it is myth. It does require institutional commitment. It does require being sensitive to both culture and language and the other things that our panel have appropriate already shared with you.

But it can be done and we have been able to do it and we have been able to demonstrate how well it can occur. And it is occurring in the California context. And California has come a long way, because 15 years ago California was doing a lousy job. But that has changed significantly.

The CHAIRMAN. You would say that in 15 years you have seen that?

Dr. ODEN. Yes, sir.

Senator PACKWOOD. Is part of it—and it is funny that he is sitting in the same chair Dr. Schultze was sitting in. And Dr. Schultze says there is no indemnity left in Southern California. It is all—he even talked about the spot market for what kind of operation?

The CHAIRMAN. Bone marrow.

Senator PACKWOOD. Bone marrow. You have a contract that will pay you $80,000 to do it and they will come and say we have one, will you do it for $60,000.

Could this be a factor that California has so long been an HMO market that you are more experienced than the rest of the country in serving people in that kind of a situation?

Dr. ODEN. That is correct. It is a more mature market. The penetration by managed care organizations is much larger. Institutions, both hospitals, as well as managed care organizations, as well as providers, have learned how to work in this competitive context and we are seeing a different set of behavior now in the context of Los Angeles and California than we are seeing in the rest of the country.

You can come to California and see the future because we have been there longer.

The CHAIRMAN. Now, now. [Laughter.]

Senator PACKWOOD. We will soon be able to see it in rural Virginia.

Dr. ODEN. Right. [Laughter.]

The CHAIRMAN. Mr. McCabe?

Mr. MCCABE. Well, I do not know if New York is in the middle of between Rhode Island and California on the map but I think one of the difficulties we have is that a lot of the terms we use mean different things to different people. I think if you talk about primary care and managed care and health care networks, if you talk to 10 people you might get 13 different opinions.

I think in some sense I would agree with both. I think that if you look at the New York experience we do not have Medicaid managed care programs that really work now. I think we are just going through the understanding that in order to make them work the institutions have to change and also the patients themselves have to change.

They have to change. They cannot show up in the emergency room when they want to. They have to keep appointments. They have to understand that they have to take care of themselves better.

But on the other hand, I do think that you could, with a committed staff of people, some infrastructure development, a good computer system to access data, I think you could have an efficient managed care program in New York. In fact, that is what we are trying to get to.

The CHAIRMAN. I would just like to note for the record that Dr. Oden's response to Senator Packwood's remark was mysterious, they are thinking of opening a new Disney World over across the way in Virginia. That is what he meant.

I do note that Dr. Smith and Dr. Oden are both from California.

Dr. SMITH. I think that is significant. Because as I said, while this varies around the country,there is no question that the trend is toward the kind of mature managed care markets that one sees in California, Minnesota and other parts of the country.

The CHAIRMAN. And Minnesota, about which we have heard a good deal.

Senator Chafee?

Senator CHAFEE. Thank you very much, Mr. Chairman.

First, I want to commend Dr. Smith. We have had quotes here from Theodore Roosevelt, and Mother Theresa, and even Yogi Beara. But this is the first time since I have been on this committee that Machiavelli has been quoted. [Laughter.]

It is really a good one. I suppose maybe Machiavelli is like the Bible, if you look long enough you can probably find a pretty good quote in there. But I find this an excellent one, which I plan to appropriate, perhaps without giving you full credit, Doctor.

Dr. SMITH. Certainly. [Laughter.]

I am certainly in no position to take credit for Machiavelli. [Laughter.]

Senator CHAFEE. But I like it. "The luke warm tempered pot rises partly from the fear of adversaries who have the laws on their side and partly from the incredulity of mankind who will never admit the merit of anything new." Let me see if I can work that into my——[Laughter.]

I want to say that I found this a very, very helpful panel, Mr. Chairman. I think the points that each of the witnesses have brought up have been good. They are right there. I suppose no hospital is more in the middle of it than Dr. McCabe's hospital. And certainly Dr. Oden and Dr.Stanley Block are right down there on the firing line as I previously mentioned.

I think that each have cited the problems as they see them. And it may be the difference between California and Rhode Island is the familiarity with the community health centers and working within them. But I certainly am very aware of all the points that Dr. Block has made and the problems he has encountered, giving specific references thereto.

I am deeply disturbed, Mr. Chairman, about the inability of our State and the community health centers to reach an agreement on a managed care waiver.

Doctor, I spoke yesterday with the Governor, Governor Sunland, on this very matter to see if they cannot reach this agreement, which I understood Friday evening they were close to, but then it fell apart. So I will keep plugging on that to try and work on this problem. It is so important to our citizens.

I also want to say, Mr. Chairman, I thought the final point that Dr. Block made about illegal aliens is a good one. That is a sensitive problem. I think that it is one that if you poll our citizens, clearly they are disturbed over the care given to illegal aliens.

I have seen some statistics on the cost in Los Angeles. They are shocking. But then the question is, "what do you do?" What do you do when a woman shows up in Dr. Block's community health center——

The CHAIRMAN. You treat her.

Senator CHAFEE. And you say, first of all, one of the virtues of their community health centers, they do not ask whether you are an illegal alien. They have no questions like that, because once they started down that path, they would frighten away the patients that have to be served.

So this is a very, very difficult problem and Dr. Block has pointed out that not only failure to treat to these individuals—it is not solely the pregnant woman that is there on your doorstep, but it is the youngster that might have some communicable disease that could affect the other children in the neighborhood who are not illegal aliens.

So it is a very, very difficult problem. I tend toward the care for them and then wrestle with the situation later on.

The CHAIRMAN. Of course you do.

Senator CHAFEE. I just do not think you can say, "well, you cannot prove your legal status here so we are not going to treat you." It is a difficult problem.

I want to thank all the panelists. I thought they were excellent.

The CHAIRMAN. Thank you, Senator Chafee.

Could I make a point, about which I am not sure I am absolutely on solid ground? I think the idea of an illegal alien is about 70 years old in the United States, is it not?

Senator CHAFEE. Well, you are the historian on this. [Laughter.]

But I have said frequently, Mr. Chairman, that one of the virtues of serving on this committee with you that I have received a Harvard education for no tuition sought. [Laughter.]

The CHAIRMAN. And like most Harvard educations, they are given by people who went to CCNY. [Laughter.]

Just to pause a moment on that, until 1924 with some interim legislation in 1916, anybody who wanted to come into the United States just came. We began to check for typhus and things like that in the 1890's. But you did not need any passport. In 1914, two countries of the world had passports. Russia and Bulgaria were the only two countries in the world that required passports.

You could get a passport if you wanted to show it around and say the Secretary of State said to be nice to this fellow, he is a big fellow in Kansas, as is our next distinguished questioner. Sir. [Laughter.]

Senator CHAFEE. And he is a big fellow in Kansas.

Senator DOLE. Kansas, right.

Well, in any event, I certainly appreciate this. I have had a chance to read the statements I did not hear earlier, part of Drs. Block and Smith. I was in L.A. recently and we had a couple of hours to sit around and talk about health care with a lot of people, so I missed you two.

But when you stop and think about L.A. County with 9 million people, as they told me it was more population than 42 of our States, they have a real problem in L.A. County—3 million people without any coverage; 1 million illegals, at least that is the estimate. Maybe that is overstated according to Dr. Delgado.

It has to put an enormous burden on hospitals and on the welfare system and on schools. But I must say, they indicated, at least as I recall, that there was not really that much abuse of the system. Even the people who sought care were not there every day or abusing the system and particularly the older people who did not have the coverage.

But according to Dr. Delgado, is that an overstatement of the problem? How do you deal with a million illegals? It is going to be a big issue. When it comes to the Senate floor, maybe even before, there is going to be a lot of debate whether we provide emergency care and send them back to wherever they are from.

If you watched the piece of 60 Minutes how they had it all planned. When the pregnant mother arrived at the hospital it was too late to send them back. How are we going to deal with the problem and just say that you just take care of it. Maybe that is the answer. I think there will be a very active debate on this one issue, even though overall—what did you say—1.6 percent of the population?

Dr. DELGADO. 1.6 percent of the U.S. population is undocumented. First of all, I am not an immigration person; I am a health person. I care about the health of Hispanics and everyone else because we all live in a community. I would say to focus on health.

You know, one thing about being undocumented is that you do not want to come face to face with government systems if you are not here legally. So the idea that these people are going to come in and get services is not consistent with an idea of being an undocumented person. What you want to do is stay away from services.

I think what we are concerned about, the emergency services will have to be provided to anybody because that is what you get throughout the world. But what most of the health care proposals would do is knock people out of the preventive services, the prevention information, those kinds of things which are relatively inexpensive and which really protect the health of a whole community.

I think we have to look at our communities as people who live there. If there is an immigration problem, you know, handle it some place else, but not in health because that affects everybody else. It is unfortunate that our media is so irresponsible in what they show in that they pull the emotional strings without having the facts behind them.

In fact, if you look at Mexican mothers who have their babies in the U.S., most of them, if they do, go to a mid—wife, pay for it out of cash, and do not end up in the emergency rooms. Because if you do, you are going to have to meet with those legal systems.

So it is like, you say, oh, these people are using services, but most of these people when they are here are avoiding interacting with the government, plus they are working. They pay taxes. They pay all sorts of sales taxes, real estate taxes by the rent and all sorts of things that they do. I think you have to look at it in both ways. It is not a simple issue and it should not be defined under health.

I used to be in HHS, and in 1981 I staffed Surgeon General Koop's task force looking at what happened with undocumented persons. At that time Secretary Schweichter was saying, oh, big problem, big problem with all these people. And the Department discovered that when they looked at Social Security applicants who had lied about their ethnicity or country of origin most to get benefits they were Canadians. And if you think about it, it makes sense.

It is much harder for someone who looks like me, who does not speak English, to say oh, I am really an American than for someone else. So I think we have to look a lot more carefully at this whole issue and understand health, it is different.

Senator DOLE. Does everybody agree with the term essential community providers, what that includes? Have you looked that up in Websters and it tells you what that is?

The CHAIRMAN. Or our lexicon.

Senator DOLE. Or a lexicon, because I want to ask about community empowerment model, too, whatever that is. But there is fair agreement on essential community providers?

Dr. SMITH. I think so. I am not sure we agree exactly on who they ought to be or how they ought to be handled. But I think everyone is agreed that there is a class of providers who have traditionally provided care for the poor who deserve some special attention as health care reform goes forward.

Senator DOLE. Can you merge that with managed care? Is that a problem?

Mr. McCABE. No, I do not think it is. I think what we are afraid of, to a certain degree, is that when you have universal coverage or everyone has a card or they all have access to the system different than they have now, that a lot of the other—the for-profit companies, HMOs, and others—will come in and then want to take care of this population.

Assuming that something changed dramatically, then they would leave and then the care would not be provided in this long term way. What we are saying is that maybe the best way to deal with these unforeseen consequences is to build upon the system that exists today.

Dr. ODEN. Senator Dole, in our health delivery system there are three community health centers that, in fact, are part of the 70 medical organizations that are part of our HMO. They serve our patients extremely well. Our patients are very satisfied with the services. And community health centers clearly are one of the leaders in serving underserved communities.

The question is really, just how do you address the involvement? In what ways can community health centers best participate in the changed environment or changing environment? I think that is where there may be a difference in emphasis, but certainly not a difference in the importance of these providers.

Dr. SMITH. Senator Dole, since I do not represent either side of this debate from the standpoint of a provider, perhaps I can just draw out what I think is the nub of the difference. I think that people who work in public hospitals, community health centers, public clinics, and other traditional centers are concerned that big, well-organized, usually insurance company backed plans will now see a market they are interested in that they were not interested in before.

They are better organized. They are better trained. They are better capitalized. They will be more attractive in some ways. And they are afraid that the traditional providers will get swamped. So they argue, if you are going to do business in Harlem, you have to contract with my hospital. It sounds reasonable.

On the other side, you have heard Dr. Oden say, and I think it is indisputable, if plans are to be held accountable for quality and for price, they have to in turn hold their providers accountable.

You cannot say to me if I am a plan operator that on the one hand I have to deliver the goods of a certain quality at a certain price and on the other that I must take any provider who shows up at my door.

So there are the two conflicting viewpoints and I think there are arguments to be made on both sides. But forgive me if I have vulgarized it, but my sense is that those are the two points of view that you hear represented here.

Mr. MCCABE. But I do think, Senator, that the issue of quality has to be sacra sync in everyone's view. I do not think that the doctors—and we are talking about making up networks for physicians that have been there for a long time, and health centers, and hospitals.

We have a private hospital ourselves but we have been there for a long time. I think that sometimes what happens is, the specter of quality is introduced as though what goes on in these neighborhoods is not quality. I think what we are talking about is creating standards that are understood and agreed upon by everyone so the playing field is level.

But there has to be some kind of access to a sort of capital base in order to make this happen.

Dr. DELGADO. I get concerned when people think that what people are asking for is for high technology and those kinds of things. That is not necessarily what we are talking about.

A good example is to look at what happens with women's health. Women go in to get care having the same symptoms as men; and yet, if they have heart disease, they are much less likely to get the appropriate treatment. That speaks to the quality of care and that is not necessarily something that has to do with high tech equipment, but just are they getting the right diagnosis, the right treatment plans.

So when you talk about quality, it would be very sad if what you measured were very concrete things and not those things that have to do with actual outpatient outcome.

Dr. BLOCK. And if I could just add that from the community health center perspective, I would disagree just a little bit with the gentleman to my right in that I do not think we are asking that HMOs be required to contract with all provides in the inner city.

I think what we are saying is that those providers that have a demonstrated commitment over a quarter of a century, that have had enormous quality assurance efforts which are required by the Federal Government's HHS, that those providers whose physicians have wanted to serve there, they are not serving there because of the bottom line, they are not serving over the past quarter of a century because they could not get jobs elsewhere. They are serving there because that is their commitment.

I think it is very important that plans be required to contract with such organizations, but not every and all organizations. I think it is very dangerous to say that a well-financed, well-capitalized HMO can come in displace the very committed providers at your site, at ours, and then in a year or two who knows whether they will still be there.

Frankly, they have not shown a very good record over the past quarter century of being so committed to the inner city poor. I think it has been quite the opposite, Senator.

Dr. DELGADO. And with all due respect to the gentleman from Los Angeles, 23 percent of the people from California are Hispanic and a lot of them are in L.A. Now I am talking as someone from Brooklyn. To me California is not the panacea. [Laughter.]

But our members at COSSMHO who are in L.A., our people are underserved. So there is a miss. So, again, you know, we have the same information but different outcomes.

Dr. ODEN. Well, I am not sure there is necessarily a miss. There are not enough providers. I think we would all agree with that. I would think also that in terms of again the issue of entitling participation has to come with some accountability also.

Community health centers have an excellent and a wonderful record of serving inner city areas. But any class of provider that is entitled and at the same time is not held to current responsibilities creates a problem. Because as you found with any group of employees who cannot be fired, they do not perform the same way as those in which they know they have to continue to perform.

It is not a knock on community health centers. It is just part of any human behavior. Entitlement in and of itself does not necessarily assure continued responsibility.

The CHAIRMAN. Mr. McCabe, you wanted to make the last statement.

Mr. MCCABE. Governor Cuomo has a Health Care Advisory Committee and the Commissioner of Health, Dr. Chassen, has been working for about 5 years trying to define outcomes with the issue of measuring quality. It has been a very difficult process.

I think that it is easy in some way to say that we are going to measure quality and the profit making plans and others are going to bring quality into the mix. But I think that we have to get a definition of precisely what quality is, what outcomes mean, before we can say it is not the case.

The CHAIRMAN. And I believe we have had a fair amount of testimony that this is an emerging methodology, if you want to use as dry a term as that. People are thinking about it. You are talking about it.

Thank you, Senator Dole.

Senator Durenberger?

Senator DURENBERGER. I will pass, Mr. Chairman. Thank you.

The CHAIRMAN. Senator Pryor?

Senator PRYOR. Thank you, Mr. Chairman. I am going to also pass. But I would like to submit a statement for the record.

The CHAIRMAN. Please do.

[The prepared statement of Senator Pryor appears in the appendix.]

Senator PRYOR. For the upcoming panel I may have some questions.

The CHAIRMAN. Thank you, sir.

Senator Conrad?

Senator CONRAD. I will pass, too. Thank you.

The CHAIRMAN. I would like to say to our distinguished witnesses that there is an urban/rural divide in our Nation and nothing seems to change it.

Before you leave though, I want to read that last passage from Machiavelli, I do not know if to give heart, but to give notice to Senator Chafee who has a very important bill before this committee.

It says that, "Whenever the enemies of change make an attack they do so with all the zeal of partisans. All the others defend themselves so feebly as to endanger both themselves and their cause." Be warned. [Laughter.]

Thank you very much. You could not have been more helpful. You have taught us things we did not know and helped us understand things we have been hearing. We very much appreciate it.

Now, can we ask our next panel to impanel itself. We have Mr. Walter Busch, who is the administrator of the Roosevelt Memorial Medical Center at Culbertson, MT; Mr. Orlo Dietrich, executive vice president of CoreSource of Chicago; Dr. Heidi Hartmann, who is the director of the Institute for Women's Policy Research here in Washington. It is nice to see you, Dr. Hartmann. Bernard Simmons, who is the executive director of the Southwest Health Agency for Rural People of Tylertown, MS, Mr. Simmons; and Edward

Ullmann of the WellCare Management Group, which I am happy to report is located in Kingston, NY, but is active in more than one State.

Just one second. Senator Baucus wants to introduce you, sir. He is on his way.

Senator DOLE. Mr. Chairman?

The CHAIRMAN. Sir.

Senator DOLE. Could I just indicate, I am afraid I am going to have to miss this panel. I am supposed to offer an amendment at 11:30 on the floor. I am certain that Senator Conrad, and Senator Pryor and others of us from rural areas will cover it well. I want to apologize to the panel for missing their testimony.

The CHAIRMAN. Well, thank you very much for coming. It has been a day when you have 1,000 places to be and things to do. All of this will be on the record and you have the testimony anyway.

Senator PRYOR. Mr. Chairman, may I make a statement while we are waiting on Senator Baucus? I, too, may have to be leaving shortly and I certainly did want to hear this panel and I have several questions if we could keep the record open for a few days.

The CHAIRMAN. The record will be open.

[The questions appear in the appendix.]

Senator PRYOR. While I do not know him well enough to really give an introduction, I wish to note that one of our panelists, Mr. Dietrich, now of Chicago, we continue to claim as an Arkansan. We hope that you still claim us.

Mr. DIETRICH. Thank you.

Senator PRYOR. Mr. Dietrich, thank you.

The CHAIRMAN. Well, that got off to a good start there. And now we will begin the panel, as I noted, Senator Baucus was anxious to introduce our first witness, Mr. Busch, of Culbertson, Montana.

Senator BAUCUS. Thank you very much, Mr. Chairman. You are correct, I am very honored to introduce Mr. Busch. Mr. Busch is the administrator of a very important facility demonstrating a very important concept, that is medical assistance facilities.

I think that these facilities are the best way to provide rural care in a facility in very rural areas. We are proud in Montana. This is a concept that we pioneered and Walter is one of the pioneers in Culbertson.

Culbertson is over in the far eastern part of our State. There are not a lot of people in Culbertson, but it is people that are very proud. I must say, Mr. Chairman, when I have attended the dedications of the openings of medical assistance facilities, like the one in Culbertson—we have two or three in Montana—I am amazed at the number of people who are there.

There are more people who come to these openings than there are people who reside in all our surrounding counties because they are so appreciative that they have a facility here, something they can be proud of that works. I am very honored that Walter is here because he has done one heck of a good job and a wonderful service.

The CHAIRMAN. Well, the more then do we look forward to your testimony, sir.

STATEMENT OF WALTER S. BUSCH, ADMINISTRATOR, ROOSEVELT MEMORIAL MEDICAL CENTER, CULBERTSON, MT

Mr. BUSCH. Thank you, Senator Baucus and Senator Moynihan. I am honored to be here. A medical assistance facility represents a unique approach to providing health care in remote areas. I can say very clearly that if the medical assistance facility model was not in place, our facility would have closed for acute care services at least 12 months ago.

At the time we made our conversion we were on the verge of closure. In fact, many other medical assistance facilities that in place in Montana were closed and reopened as a result of the medical assistance facility model.

It has some unique characteristics that are suited to frontier areas. Perhaps the most important in our experience has been the better utilization of physician extenders—mid-level practitioners such as physician assistants or nurse practitioners.

Under the MAF regulations, the MAF allows the mid—levels to admit patients, take emergency room call, to provide a much wider array of services. We have had tremendous difficulty recruiting primary care physicians in rural Montana, partly because of the lower volumes. We have a diverse population scattered over a large geographic area.

It is difficult to have more than one physician in many of these towns. One physician tends to burn out if they are taking call 24 hours a day, 7 days a week.

Under the MAF model we have ended up now with two extenders, two physicians assistants and one physician, all of whom rotate call.

The CHAIRMAN. Mr. Busch, we keep working on a lexicon around here. Senator Packwood knows what a physician assistant is. I do not. Would you give us a little more information? Nurse practitioner is a familiar term. Physician assistant.

Mr. BUSCH. Physician assistants have a different training module. I believe the concept of the profession evolved out of the medics from the Vietnam War. Instead of going through nurse training, some of those individuals became involved in programs that led to physician assistant categorization.

In terms of what they do, it is equivalent to nurse practitioners, but it does not go through the nurse training.

The CHAIRMAN. All right.

Mr. BUSCH. They are specialists in surgery as physician assistants and OB/GYN and primary care.

Both of these used the medical assistance models very effectively. The physician assistant by law has to be linked to a supervising physician. In our case, if a physician assistant makes an admission to the MAF, a physician has to be notified within 24 hours of that admission. The nurse practitioner is more independent under the law.

I was reviewing our financial reports just before I came out here. Another important fact of MAF is that it is cost based reimbursement under the old system, where we are reimbursed reasonable costs for providing the service. We are not under the perspective payment DRG system.

In a small low-volume facility, that is very important. As a perspective based facility prior to MAF, we were losing a great deal of money. Now going into our second year, it looks like we will be running probably about $2,000 to the good. It is about an $80,000 turnaround in terms of bottom line.

At the same time, our expenses are declining. The MAF model is a very flexible model and it allows not only communities to design the facility around their needs, but also the facility itself to be very flexible as to how it provides care.

We have more flexibility in terms of the mid-level practitioner and in terms of nurse coverage. We have been involved in a great deal of cross training in our facility since becoming an MAF and our expense levels are down about $200,000 which in a $2 million budget that is relatively significant.

So even though we are cross based, we find that we can run much more efficiently now than we could before and it is having an affect on the cost of providing a service.

We have also transitioned with assistance of some grants to largely primary care, preventive health, wellness. We have the WIC program, Meals-on-Wheels. We have well child immunizations, plus general acute and emergency room services.

This is said to increase networking with other facilities in our area. So it leads to an informal networking, which I think leads to a higher quality of care for all concerned.

We serve primarily Medicare patients, just because of our demographic situation, and it works really well for that. What we have not addressed with the MAF and which I hope can be addressed by Congress is access for everyone. We find in our communities, I would say the vast majority have no health insurance because they cannot afford it.

Our employees, we reimburse 75 percent of the cost of health insurance for employees themselves. We are pat of a six hospital group to try and hold our insurance costs down. We have gone from a $300 deductible to a $1,000 deductible this past year and even so our rates have gone up 50 percent, to the point where I am not sure how much longer we can afford it.

The school system in Culbertson now provides—I believe it is $200 per employee, rather than provide health insurance because of the cost of health insurance. I think we are pretty typical of Montana. I think the vast major, the big majority of people have no health insurance and simply cannot afford it.

In my written testimony I included some information from the U.S. Department of Commerce about average salaries. I think in our State it is about $18,000. Although the cost of living is lower in rural areas, the cost of a car is the same; the cost of clothes is the same. About the only benefit you have is the cost of housing. Food is actually more expensive; transportation is more expensive because you are traveling 50 to 100 miles to go shopping very often.

So that access to coverage is protected through models such as the MAF, but getting everybody to be able to use them, we have not solved that problem yet. Nearer the views of speakers earlier argued for universal coverage. I think that is really important however that be provided. Probably if it is mandated through employer participation then we would need subsidies because many of our limited employment opportunities are not making very much money either.

But as I say, most do not provide any benefits in terms of health insurance. This is the main reason I am here today is to just share our positive experience as an MAF. It is a demonstration project.

HCFA and the Montana State Health Department have played a large role in making it successful. Senator Baucus has been a key player in helping us survive in the last 5 years.

We think in Montana, those of us that are MAFs, that it is worthy of inclusion as a permanent part of Medicare and that it should be open to other frontier areas in the country. It is relatively simple to operate. It does not have a lot of bureaucratic rules, but it is very effective. We find it to be very cost effective.

The quality reviews we have done on a State wide basis are very good. When patients require transfer to a higher level of facility they are transferred. We have improved communication with large facilities. I think it is a model worthy of inclusion on a national level. Thank you very much.

The CHAIRMAN. We thank you, sir.

[The prepared statement of Mr. Busch appears in the appendix.]

Senator GRASSLEY. Mr. Chairman?

The CHAIRMAN. Senator?

Senator GRASSLEY. Could I have 60 seconds, please?

The CHAIRMAN. You can have as much time as you want.

Senator GRASSLEY. The bankruptcy bill is up on the floor and I am the Republican manager on that.

I will take 60 seconds now and I will read their answer in the transcript. But several of them could be concerned about the Medicare dependent hospital program. And specifically, Mr. Simmons, I know, makes mention of it in his statement. I think in Mississippi there are 24 such hospitals. That programs ends October of this year, Mr. Chairman.

When we developed that legislation which called for the ending of that program at that time, we assumed that there would be a simultaneous phaseout of the urban/rural differential and that it would make up the financial loss so that the hospitals would not have the financial problems that brought about a Medicare dependent program in the first place.

I would like to ask the people on the panel how they see the phaseout of the medicare dependent hospital program affecting them. We are not seeing the rural/urban wage differential phaseout make up that money that was in the Medicare dependent hospital program.

We are going to lose in my State a lot of money when the program expires in October. It might be difficult for them to survive without that help. I am interested in finding out from the panel—and I will read the answers in the transcript—whether the consequences would be the same in these other States. And particularly, I am interested in Mississippi since Mr. Simmons mentions that.

I suppose the bottom line is, what is the situation when the program ends in October in your specific State.

The CHAIRMAN. Mr. Simmons, if you have a moment, Senator Grassley.

Senator GRASSLEY. I can wait. I did not want to take the time of the committee though.

The CHAIRMAN. This is your committee, too.

Senator GRASSLEY. All right. Thank you.

Mr. SIMMONS. We recommend from the National Health Association that Medicare dependent hospitals be considered the class of essential community providers as well which is protected as the central providers. The wage differential has not been erased and is one of the things that we are concerned with, the biases that come forth in health care reform that they do not perpetuate the same thing that has happened in the past.

Senator GRASSLEY. And you would find that the financial situation would—in other words, the money lost from the Medicare dependent hospital program is not made up by the rural/urban differential phaseout?

Mr. SIMMONS. It is not.

Senator GRASSLEY. Thank you.

Mr. SIMMONS. In our case we run the risk of losing our admitting hospital——

The CHAIRMAN. So we have something to deal with by October 1.

Senator GRASSLEY. Well, from my standpoint I think yes and also from Senator Dole's standpoint. I think to some extent Minnesota. But there is more than just a handful of States that are affected.

The CHAIRMAN. Senator Baucus indicated he would. Would that be the case, Mr. Busch?

Mr. BUSCH. We are on cost-based reimbursement. But I would say that is the case for rural Montana, yes.

The CHAIRMAN. Well,thank you, Senator Grassley. If you want to have written questions, we will get written answers.

Senator GRASSLEY. Thank you.

The CHAIRMAN. And now Mr. Dietrich, we welcome you, sir, as the executive vice president of CoreSource in Chicago.

STATEMENT OF ORLO L. DIETRICH, JR., EXECUTIVE VICE PRESIDENT, CORESOURCE, INC., CHICAGO, IL

Mr. DIETRICH. Mr. Chairman and members of the committee, thank you for the opportunity to appear at this important hearing today. My name is Orlo Dietrich and I am the executive vice president of CoreSource, a national managed care and information company that developed and manages rural based managed care delivery systems.

Our company has over the past 10 years developed 175 of these networks in 31 States, serving over 300,000 people.

The written statement, which I have submitted for the record, frames many of the fundamental reform issues being debated within the contexts of our experiences in rural America. Today in my oral remarks the central message I bring is that private sector managed health care can work in rural America and it can effectively address the key reform issues relating to cost containment, universal coverage, patient access and quality medical care.

For the past 10 years our company has witnessed the evolution and growth of private sector solutions to rural health care delivery, solutions that can flourish under reform legislation.

Eleven years ago I was an employer in Mount Home, Arkansas with responsibility for over 3,000 manufacturing employees in a community of under 10,000. Additionally, I served as a Board trustee for the local hospital and knew many of the physicians.

Our concerns then—this is 1984—were many of the same that exist today—the employer's concern over escalating cost. The hospital strove to maintain its financial viability in the face of the unnecessary out migration of medical dollars to the larger communities. Physicians struggling with the issues of physician recruitment and patient access. And everyone committed to protecting and enhancing the availability of quality medical care for the community.

The nucleus of that local community in 1984 formed the nucleus of the model which now serves all of our programs nationally. Specifically, a community health plan driven by a nonadversarial relationship between the payers and providers focused around a local government structure which continually addresses the effective utilization of medical services by both patients and medical provides.

Ten years and 175 communities later the same fundamentals still apply. What has changed and changed dramatically is the pace at which these initiatives are sweeping rural America and the forces behind these changes.

Until approximately 1992 the great majority of rural health care initiatives, while supported by the medical communities, were initiated by the private sector in an effort to control cost.

Today the national reform debate has driven home the reality that regardless of the outcome of reform, rural health care will become managed health care. The acceptance of this reality has driven rural medical communities to begin searching for solutions which will allow providers to maintain some control over their future and to protect them from the large subordinate role they fear when a large insurance entity or a metropolitan hospital begins carving up the geography with little concern for the long term viability of the smaller community.

As rural providers have searched for solutions, they have recognized that private sector employers are their strongest supporters. While there is the honest recognition that each group has its own vested concerns, there is the stronger belief that each is a dependent part of a somewhat fragile hole, a rural community. And this sense of community often missing in urban areas creates the willingness to work cooperatively together for effective and long term solution.

Our strong belief is that while systematic health care reform is clearly needed, it must recognize and address the fragile and unique nature of rural America and effectively support local communities as they work together developing local solutions.

Clearly, we must recognize that for many of these communities any mandate for competitive programs would fatally fracture the local medical delivery system. We must also recognize that private employers within these communities are vital to these efforts.

Without the involvement and commitment of the private sector employers, the necessary balance between payers and providers will not exist.

Again, I appreciate the opportunity to speak and hope that my comments you will not only appreciate the uniqueness of our rural communities, but view them not as problems in a reform debate, but as models producing real solutions.

Thank you very much.

The CHAIRMAN. We thank you, sir.

[The prepared statement of Mr. Dietrich appears in the appendix.]

The CHAIRMAN. You have 50 of these in Arkansas alone, do you not?

Senator PRYOR. Yes.

The CHAIRMAN. This is something we will turn to with questioning. We much appreciate that, indeed.

We are going to hear now from Dr. Hartmann, who is well known to our committee, on behalf of the Institute for Women's Policy Research. Welcome again.

STATEMENT OF HEIDI I. HARTMANN, PH.D., DIRECTOR, INSTITUTE FOR WOMEN'S POLICY RESEARCH, WASHINGTON, DC

Dr. HARTMANN. Thank you. I am Heidi Hartmann, director of the Institute for Women's Policy Research. I am a labor economist and hold the Ph.D. degree from Yale University. I want to thank you, Chairman Moynihan and members of the committee, for the opportunity to testify here today.

It is a pleasure to share our new research findings with you at this important hearing on underserved populations in health care reform. My testimony today addresses the needs of another underserved population—women—and it is based on our forthcoming report on women's access to health insurance, viewing health insurance as the first step in access to actually getting health care.

It presents findings from the first thorough study of the factors that affect women's access and lack of access to health insurance. Our forthcoming report also assesses how well President Clinton's proposed Health Security Act would address women's needs.

Our study was conducted by a team of five IWPR researchers, many of whom are here with me today, that relies on data collected.

The CHAIRMAN. Could I just ask if you might introduce them.

Dr. HARTMANN. I would love to.

The CHAIRMAN. Dr. Young-Hee Yoon.

Dr. HARTMANN. Yes, Dr. Young-Hee Yoon is here right behind me.

The CHAIRMAN. Stand up. Come on now. There you are.

Dr. HARTMANN. Dr. Young-Hee Yoon is a sociologist.

The CHAIRMAN. Good morning, Doctor.

Dr. HARTMANN. Dr. Lois Shaw is an economist.

The CHAIRMAN. Good morning, Doctor.

Dr. HARTMANN. Stephanie Aaronson.

The CHAIRMAN. Ms. Aaronson, the committee welcomes you.

Dr. HARTMANN. And Dr. Spalter-Roth is not with us this morning.

The CHAIRMAN. We welcome her in absentia.

Dr. HARTMANN. Well, I think you know her well in our welfare reform debates.

The CHAIRMAN. That is right.

Dr. HARTMANN. I would like to point out that our study is based on Census Bureau data from the current population survey. This is a survey of 60,000 households taken every month and it is representative of the nation's population as a whole. The study was funded by the Henry F. Kaiser Family Foundation as part of their health care reform project.

We focus on women's access to health insurance for several reasons. Women have a unique relationship to the health care system in the United States that we believe needs to be taken into account in any discussion of health care reform. Women use more health care services than men and pay more for them as a proportion of their income than do men. They are also responsible for facilitating their family's access to health care and for insuring the health of infants and children.

Yet many women have no health insurance. Twelve million women of working age—18 to 64 or 15 percent of these adults—have no insurance of any kind. These women are clearly likely to be medically underserved.

I have four points in I hope about four minutes. First, it has been traditional for women to obtain health insurance indirectly through their husband's jobs, even when they themselves also work in the labor market, but this traditional system is breaking down.

More and more women are slipping through the cracks and more will continue to do so. As people marry later and divorce more, more adults are unmarried for longer portions of their lives.

Already two out of five adult women do not live with husbands, and the majority of women, even married women, do not receive their health insurance through their husband's jobs. Increasing numbers of men have jobs that do not provide health insurance, especially for other family members.

Access to dependent care coverage is falling for all workers. Given these changes taking place in family structures and employment, women have an increased need for secure access to insurance and a decreased likelihood of obtaining it through marriage. Therefore, it is important to look at how women get access to health insurance through their own employment.

Second, considering all adult women, because they are more likely than men to depend on indirect insurance through a spouse, they are at risk of losing insurance throughout the life style because of family break up. If you want to take a look at Figure 1, and I direct you toward the new figures, you can see that women have less access to health insurance through their own employers than men do—37 percent for women versus 55 percent for men.

Women have more indirect access and more public access, probably because of Medicaid and because they live longer and enjoy Medicare longer, so men have slightly less insurance overall than women do.

Women are, indeed, fortunate to have access through more sources than men, but reliance on indirect coverage through a family member leaves them vulnerable to life cycle events common to all of us, such as leaving the parental home, divorce, widowhood, or the retirement or job loss of a spouse.

Age and marital status proved even more important in our research than we thought it would. Among our most surprising findings is that young women especially lack insurance—5 million young adult women under age 30 have no insurance, yet 70 percent of births occur to women in this age group.

Women who are not married are twice as likely as married women to lack health insurance. Single mothers are also more likely to be uninsured, despite the existence of the Medicaid program which targets low-income single mothers and their children.

As other researchers have found, race, low educational attainment and low family income are all associated with lack of insurance. Over 4 million women of color lack insurance.

The third point, employed women hold marginal places in the labor market and so obtain less employer provided insurance directly. But they also have less coverage when they work in similar jobs as men.

You might be particularly interested in the coverage rates in agriculture since you are interested in rural issues. They are especially low in agriculture. Only 21 percent of women and 23 percent of men have coverage that comes from their own employer. And interestingly, very interestingly, indirect coverage through spouses employment is also exceptionally low, likely reflecting the lack of alternative types of employment in rural areas that could provide access to health insurance corroborating your point.

You might want to look at Figure 2 and Tables 2A and B.

Fourth, close to the final point, I believe.

The CHAIRMAN. Take your time.

Dr. HARTMANN. Plenty of time?

The CHAIRMAN. Yes.

Dr. HARTMANN. Our findings on the impact of the Health Security Act, particularly the employer mandate that would require all employers to contribute to health insurance for workers who work at least 10 hours per week shows striking results, especially for the uninsured and I will focus just on the results for the uninsured here in my oral presentation.

Figure 3 displays some of those results. The following would gain coverage directly from their own employers for the first time and not all these numbers are on your figure. I apologize for that, but you cannot get them all on.

Eight million uninsured working women and 12 million uninsured working men or three-quarters of all the uninsured adults would be covered under this type of employer mandate; 6 million uninsured women, earning less than $12,000 annually, and 7 million uninsured men earning at the same level, in other words the low earners would particularly benefit from the mandate in terms of gaining access to insurance; 3 million uninsured women working in large firms, those with 100 or more employees, and 4 million similar situated men. In other words, this is not just a small firm problem, this is also a large firm problem.

In particular, there are a million women working in large firms in the retail trade that do not get insurance. Also, there are 2.5 million uninsured men working in construction firms, mostly in small firms, and all of these also would get insurance through the type of employer mandate that is specified in President Clinton's plan.

Finally, if the size of the firm that were subject to the mandate were changed—in President Clinton's plan it is all employers—if it were changed to that those with fewer than 25 employees were dropped from the employer mandate provision, we found that the proportion of the uninsured who would gain health insurance would fall from three-quarters of all the uninsured to only two-fifths. And if you increase the size of the exemption to 200, the number covered would fall to one-quarter, a substantial decrease.

In conclusion, our study shows that reform that includes an employer mandate would address many of the problems in health insurance access that women currently have. Having direct access to insurance through their own employer would protect many women from losing insurance as the result of reaching adulthood, family break up due to divorce or separation or the job loss of the insured through retirement or unemployment.

Having greater access to insurance from their own employers would thus provide greater security to women undergoing transitions in their family arrangements. Also, under the Health Security Act, which goes beyond an employer mandate by also guaranteeing universal access and through providing cost subsidies, workers do not have to fear loss of insurance when they change jobs, experience unemployment or leave the labor market for a period of time.

However, even with the Health security Act there are certainly some issues of concern for men such as the fact that if you have low earnings the cost sharing that you would have to do as a worker might be relatively high for you. You might experience it as high. And, of course, women do have lower earnings and lower incomes than men on average.

Thank you.

The CHAIRMAN. Thank you, Dr. Hartmann, once again.

[The prepared statement of Dr. Hartmann appears in the appendix.]

The CHAIRMAN. And now Mr. Simmons on behalf of the National Rural Health Association.

STATEMENT OF BERNARD SIMMONS, EXECUTIVE DIRECTOR, SOUTHWEST HEALTH AGENCY FOR RURAL PEOPLE, INC., AND MEMBER, BOARD OF TRUSTEES, NATIONAL RURAL HEALTH ASSOCIATION, TYLERTOWN, MS

Mr. SIMMONS. Thank you, Mr. Chairman and members of the Senate Finance Committee. My name is Bernard Simmons. I am a member of the Board of Trustees of the National Rural Health Association, representing what we call community operated practices, which is primarily community and migrant health centers. I am also a member of the Board of Directors of the National Association of Communities Health Centers as their Speak of the House and Chair of the Legislative Committee.

Today I am representing the National Rural Health Association, whose membership is comprised of small rural hospitals, community and migrant health centers, rural health clinics, primary care physicians, nonphysician providers, educators and other rural health advocates.

Mr. Chairman, I have submitted written testimony and request it be entered into the record.

The CHAIRMAN. Without objection.

[The prepared statement of Mr. Simmons appears in the appendix.]

Mr. SIMMONS. And would like to use the remainder of my time to highlight the impact of reform on rural underserved areas, and especially the impact on a State like Mississippi.

The National Rural Health Association urges serious consideration and passage of health care reform that ensures guaranteed universal access to primary and preventive health care services for all populations. The National Rural Health Association distinguishes universal access from universal coverage by dividing universal access as access to basic comprehensive care services.

In our estimation, providing a health care card and offering health care benefits does not go far enough to providing quality health care services. A health security card will not guarantee access to health services.

American citizens, particularly those in isolated rural and frontier communities, must have access to primary health care providers and these providers must be financially accessible with little or no co-pays and these providers must be geographically accessible, that is located in the community or less than 30 minutes driving time.

The National Rural Health Association believes that there are two major issues in financing health system reform that must be considered in implementing national health reform. These are how to finance the overall system; and, two, how to pay for services as well as reasonable costs for reimbursement, focusing on the patient provider relationship.

The National Rural Health Association recommends that reform of the health care system cannot take place by reducing Medicare. Rural areas with our disproportionate number of elderly will suffer inordinately with decrease in Medicare funding.

It is clear that historical biases in reimbursement to rural providers exist in our current system. Medicare pays rural providers up to 40 percent less than their urban counterparts for the same services. Costs for these services in rural communities are generally higher because rural providers cannot take advantage of economies of scale and many other reasons.

Therefore, the National Rural Health Association recommends that the wage index reflect the price of labor by reimbursing rural hospitals with a fair occupational mix adjustment. We further recommend in our polls, the reduction in the hospital market basket update for rural hospitals.

There are other issues around rural community based health care systems under the health care reform—federally qualified health centers, FQHCs, a term, Mr. Chairman, which you know this committee played a central role in establishing into law.

Here is an entity when which southwest health agents of our rural people is defined as an essential community provider under the President's bill. It is critical that there be a mechanism that recognize and maintain the contribution of essential community providers as community health centers and other community based providers, which have established themselves and demonstrated their ability to provide access to health care services for residents of rural underserved areas.

There must be assurances that essential community providers participate and be protected in the payment methodology agreements. Americans need more than universal coverage and comprehensive benefits. They need a health care home.

The National Rural Health Association supports cost—based reimbursement for both federally qualified health centers and rural health clinics. There is no question that bias exists in the historical payment to rural primary care providers also. The Medicare reimbursement for office visits are substantially lower than the cost of providing the services.

The National Rural Health Association is concerned about the Medicare fee schedule structure, in that while a varying geographic schedule would continue the inherent biases in restricted payments to primary care providers.

Ultimately an access problem will arise for rural residents who leave in alliances with low rates and/or high administrative costs. The National Rural Health Association believes that higher payments for primary care services can be achieved through reconfiguring the conversion factor and thus bonus payments rather than through changes in relative value.

Moreover, alliances or States should be required to adopt a national resource-based fee schedule, but allow the alliances or States to negotiate with providers regarding the conversion factor.

The National Rural Health Association supports Medicare bonus payment of increase of 20 percent for primary care providers serving in health professional shortage areas. Medicare bonus payments should continue for a period of 10 years regardless of whether the health manpower shortage designation remained in effect.

The National Rural Health Association supports the designation of essential community providers to include hospitals that qualify for a Medicare disproportionate share adjustment, federally qualified health centers, rural health clinics, sole community hospitals, hospitals that will qualify as a Medicare dependent hospital, and entities designated by the State Government through the State health plan.

The statement I make now, Mr. Chairman, is not a National Rural Health Association statement, but is a personal statement as it regards service in a State like Mississippi.

Mississippi's public policy as it relates to primary and preventive care has been lacking. I support State flexibility and State rights to develop its own health care reform. While the advantages may be many, it is important to understand the public policy approach of Mississippi's elected and appointed officials regarding the development of primary and preventive care infrastructure in the State.

Therefore, I recommend that the health care reform package assure that there are proper systems of checks and balances in place for States as they respond to the health care reform legislation, such that there is accountability by States as well.

Mississippi is very conservative fiscally and morally. Therefore, allowing States like Mississippi too much flexibility without oversight can undo and can erode advances in health care outcomes that have already been achieved thus far.

These providers have established themselves and demonstrated their ability to provide care in the underserved and underlying areas.

The last issue I wish to address with you is capital infrastructure development. There needs to be capital infrastructure development for community health centers and other community based health care institutions. Funds must be available for loans and loan guarantees, interest subsidies and direct grants.

Funding must be provided for planning and construction costs to convert existing facilities to community health centers or other community based models of care where appropriate. For example, these models would be essential community hospitals, rural primary care programs and the medical assistance facilities to name a few.

The National Rural Health Association supports funding of loans for rural health networks. However, in many isolated rural and frontier areas networks may not be possible. Therefore, it is critical that funding for capital infrastructure projects also allow for the provision of individual rural health care facilities that are community directed and accepted by the community.

In summary, I would like to recap these points. We need guarantee access to health services. That is the patient needs a medical home. A substantial commitment of resources for primary and preventive care infrastructure develop in underserved areas during the transition and after the transition occurs, a redirection of graduate medical education, funding and payment to promote primary care provider training and to allow community health centers and other essential community providers to be reimbursed for participating in training of health professionals.

Lastly, reasonable cost-based reimbursement that will assure the survival and preservation of essential community providers, like community health centers, but are the safety net for the underserved communities from unfair financial risk.

Thank you, Mr. Chairman.

The CHAIRMAN. Thank you, Mr. Simmons.

If our panel will allow a brief interruption, I would like to go into executive session at this point, as a quorum has appeared at the committee today.

[Whereupon, at 12:05 p.m., the hearing recessed and resumed at 12:07 p.m.]

The CHAIRMAN. We will now return to our regular hearing.

Concluding this morning's marvelous hearing is Edward Ullmann, who is president and chief executive officer of the WellCare Management Group, presenting an innovative and important set of ideas about this subject. We welcome you, sir, all the way down from Kingston.

Mr. ULLMANN. Your great State of New York.

STATEMENT OF EDWARD A. ULLMANN, PRESIDENT AND CHIEF EXECUTIVE OFFICER, THE WELLCARE MANAGEMENT GROUP, INC., KINGSTON, NY

Mr. ULLMANN. Thank you, Mr. Chairman and members of the committee. My formal testimony has been submitted to you.

The CHAIRMAN. We have it right here, very elegantly bound.

[The prepared statement of Mr. Ullmann appears in the appendix.]

Mr. ULLMANN. I am Ed Ullmann. I am President and CEO of WellCare. We are a 75,000 member HMO that operates in up-state New York. Our membership is a cross section of our community. It always has been heavily small business and 9,000 Medicaid recipients.

I am especially proud of the integration of the poor into our managed care systems because it is the right thing to do. We have been able to show that you can increase access and at the same time have cost containment for our governments; and most important, when they belong to the premier HMO in a community, they have dignity again when they receive health care services. We think that is very important.

Early on when we began in rural America, we realized that as an HMO we had a moral obligation to reinvest quite heavily back into the delivery system if we were going to be successful. We looked around and realized that if you did not restructure around primary care and wellness there was no shot for us to make it in rural America.

So we brought our doctors together. We sat down and said we are partners in this.

The CHAIRMAN. Now we are in Kingston, are we not?

Mr. ULLMANN. Yes, and our area is about four hours in travel distance above New York City up through Lake George.

The CHAIRMAN. And about an hour below Albany.

Mr. ULLMANN. It includes Albany and that surrounding community, too. That is correct, sir.

So we realized that the physicians were going to be the key to any long-term success and we were the insurer, we were the innovators. We had the capital to do something positive.

So we sat down with them and said, what is it that you need. What is it that we can do together? It was very interesting. They first said recruitment. So we have become the largest recruiter of providers in our community and over 22 new doctors in the last 2 years. This includes not just primary care physicians, but also the mid-level professions of nurse clinicians, and PAs that we talked about and other providers that the doctors feel that they need.

We then said what is this about burnout and how can we help. Well, we realized that the on-call coverage teams, many of these doctors were on call four or 5 days a week. Well, we organized them together so now they are on coverage maybe three times a month.

We also realized the amount of inefficiency going to the hospital every day. So we turned around and put together inpatient teams that do all the hospitalization for the doctors so they can stay in their practice and be more efficient.

We also realize there are a lot of women physicians coming in that are very concerned about quality of life issues. That is the key thing in rural America. Not economics, it is quality of life issues. And they were excellent to work at the hospitals because it allowed them to raise a family.

So we tried to be innovative and we kept saying to the doctors, what else do you need. If you are not automated, we will computerize you. If you do not want to run your practices, we will run your practices for you and you do the clinical components.

And if you keep listening to your physicians in rural America, they will stay in your communities and then you can build off of them. So we have started to develop alliances of health professionals.

Then they told me that the education to keep up was very difficult. So we put together a 120-seat lecture hall that is very much involved in continuing education programs and certification, helping the doctors to not be isolated but to communicate with each other on a regular basis.

We also realized very much that the training programs had to be a mentor type of relationship, so that the doctors who were better at managing resources can help the other physicians who are learning about it so that they can grow together and learn how to work and be successful under managed care.

We also realized that the restructuring of a delivery system was going to take guts in rural America. Everybody knows each other. It is very parochial. And you have to learn how to say no. So we realized that you had to find ways to bring a specialist and the hospitals to the risk sharing arrangements with our doctors. We have to help educate the doctors on how they can really be involved with risk sharing, limiting resources correctly without compromising on the quality of care.

That takes a lot of information systems. It takes a lot of one-on-one communications. But it can be done as WellCare has demonstrated as being a low cost provider in its community and we recently received provision accreditation by the National Committee on Quality Assurance.

So we know that you can prove quality if you really work at it and you can do it in a cost effective manner. So as we move along with the doctors we just realized that that is going to be the key solution. And as we squeeze under cost containment under any level of managed care, we are going to realize that we have over capacity and we have to be involved in the health planning of our communities so that hospitals are not scared about the loss of employment. Because we do have too many hospital beds and there is going to be a reduction of hospitals and there is going to be a reduction in a lot of the overspecialization in these communities. We cannot afford it.

I believe very much that as we move to expand the primary care delivery system around wellness we are going to have to also improve the use of alternative health providers in our communities under the supervision of primary care doctors. I am talking about chiropractors and acupuncture physicians. We need their services if we are going to continue to provide accessibility for all Americans.

I believe it can be done. We can achieve universal coverage as a basic human right in rural America, and in our urban communities, if we work together in a partnership, if we realize this is going to take us decades, if we realize that our kids require our leadership now, if we realize that medical outcomes and accountability for cost containment is going to be our future.

And most important, Mr. Chairman, if we realize that health care——

The CHAIRMAN. Medical outcomes, we have heard that 10 times this morning.

Mr. ULLMANN. Yes, over and over again.

We have to realize that health care is really the treatment of a total human being, not simply treatment of body parts. And that is going to require a whole different philosophy in this country. I think our time has come now.

Thank you very much.

The CHAIRMAN. Thank you. I think the history, is it not, that we began treating the entire human being, not very well, and then gradually learned about organs. But now there is a cycling back to knowing more about the actual system. We have started thinking in terms of that total wellness concept.

Senator Durenberger?

Senator DURENBERGER. Thank you, Mr. Chairman.

Maybe a general question of all the panelists. One of the tough issues, both with regard to the inner city and the rural areas, of course, is what we would call health, public health, community health versus access to medical services.

There is a tendency in my State, as I have noticed in many States, and to some extent here, to say well we are doing health care reform and we are going to have guaranteed access of everybody in this country to these new insurance plans called accountable health plans and we want to put all those services into those plans.

I have a hard time understanding how we do that. I cannot quite figure that out. It seems to me that a lot of the problems that plague us are environmental problems and they are different in every community in our country. I do not mean just land use, clean water and lead. I am talking about the larger behavioral and other related issues.

So maybe from the standpoint of everyone here who has looked, as all of you have, at this problem, is it even practical to think about constructing a benefit set in an accountable health plan that under the labels preventive, diagnostic, therapeutic and rehabilitative is going to right off the get go include every possible service that people working with poor, people working with those who are rationally or economically or otherwise disadvantaged, people who consistently had to live in underserved, medically underserved areas, some of the issues of the absorption of immigrants, legal and other kinds of refugees and so forth is not a simple problem to just put everybody in a health plan, then have those health plans compete and have informed consumers making choices and so forth.

I have always felt that—in fact, in a little discussion we had here on Tuesday on the so-called SIN taxes, that it is going to be a big mistake if we decide to raise the tobacco tax $2 and all the other great ideas that the Chairman has for weapons of violence and things like that, and to use that to fund access to medical services for the uninsured and leave these basic problems of kids growing up not very far to have kids themselves to have kids, to have kids, and on and on, leave all those problems to some categorical, Federal categorical, program that are not working.

I mean, the 500 or 600 programs that are designed to do some good in Mississippi are not doing any good in Minnesota because there are too many mandates to respond to the wonderful quotation from Mr. Simmons about sort of the way in which the conservative balance there. I think that is the word you used, conservative, balance their fiscal priorities and their moral priorities in a lot of areas.

So I kind of have the sense that if we go into the SIN tax business in a big way, for example, at the national level, that somehow or other we reserve some major part of that, if not all of that, to be devolved to all those communities that you all represent out there in America, to deal with the really difficult long term interrelational health problems that are not going to be solved by insurance plans or accountable health plans.

Would anybody like to make a comment on that?

Dr. HARTMANN. I would be happy to.

The CHAIRMAN. Please, Dr. Hartmann.

Dr. HARTMANN. Well, I think you are quite right about the continued even entries need for basically public health services, community health services and outreach. I think that, you know, when we talk about the savings we are going to get by having universal insurance because we think we are going to take care of health problems sooner before they get worse, et cetera, and we hope to even perhaps duplicate the savings in Canada, I think we do not realize how much a country like Canada has invested in community outreach and preventive services. They have a very much lower rate of violence, for example, than we have.

On the other hand, your other point that you are not sure that a minimum benefits package can be legislated from Washington, I would probably tend to disagree with that. I think the women's community in particular would like to see some minimum benefits guaranteed. Some of the ones that you might not have thought about as much that are relatively cheap and easy to provide and seem to be universal problems in all communities are things like domestic violence screening, screening for domestic violence as part of a minimum standard benefits package.

Senator DURENBERGER. Why would you put that in a national benefits package? Why do you not leave that to a particular health plan in a particular community? If, in fact, it is taking on some risk in that community or reducing the incidence of domestic violence so that it reduces the visits to the emergency room, the hospitals, the doctor, why do you not leave each community through their health plan to decide whether that is appropriate or not? Would that not make more sense?

Dr. HARTMANN. Well, that is certainly an alternative approach. I think that many women would find that when we have to go state-by-state or even the higher of community-by-community for certain things that we consider basic, it is very difficult.

I mean, breast cancer screening is another that women would feel very strongly about. Of course, reproductive choice is another that women feel very strongly about. So, you know, that is a philosophical difference.

Senator DURENBERGER. Yes, Mr. Dietrich.

Mr. DIETRICH. Senator, if I were to attempt to frame my answer to your question around the rural environment, I think I would divide it up a bit into the cost effective management of medical dollars and the financing of those dollars and put it all under the recognition that every community is totally different, especially in rural America. And in one community the problem is adolescent psyche and the next community the main problem may be prescription drug over usage.

We have communities where in one community there is a 55 percent Caesarean section rate and 50 miles down the road it is 22 percent. So every community has its own set of dynamics that are driving the cost escalation.

Senator DURENBERGER. Well, it is a somewhat different culture than a different way of approaching pollution.

Mr. DIETRICH. Yes, sir. There are different cultures. There are different access to health care, different levels of medical providers. Our experience has been that these communities have come to grips with their problems and have the ability to put systems together to control cost within those communities.

The thing that we have seen for the past 10 years is communities really coming to grips from both the payer and the provider perspective with how to control escalating costs. What none of us has figured out is how we do all the financing to access the people to the system. That gets us into tort reform, malpractice reform, Medicare/Medicaid reform and all of those issues that allow us to access the total patient population into delivery systems.

The good news is, these delivery systems really do control costs. They do not solve all the problems of how we finance the access to the system. But every rural community is different.

Mr. SIMMONS. I think I would agree with the previous speaker, is that I would like to see a national set of benefits, mandates or some type of a benefit package. If a plan does not have the requirement to be community responsive—and I think that is one of the beauties of community health centers around the country, they respond to the community need because they are responsible to a community board.

If the health plan does not have to provide these as a mandate for participating federally in a reform package, then they may or may not be community responsive. If it is adolescent psyche or if it domestic violence or if it is black on black crime or whatever it may be, they can be responsive to that in that health plan. But it has to be specified that you, from Washington, expects for them to be community sensitive and respond to that community need that causes the leading causes of death or disability within those communities.

Mr. ULLMANN. Senator, I would very much support that, that these integrated delivery systems competing will be successful. I think you can operate under a basic benefit package and then when outcomes technology starts to show which alternative sources of care for providers work they will incorporate them automatically as a benefit.

The CHAIRMAN. As a competitive measure.

Mr. ULLMANN. Yes, that is correct. I think outside of financing what is really needed from the national perspective is assistance with medical malpractice. I think it would be very harmful to allow each State to decide this on their own. I think also on the ethical issues and how we handle technology and what level of research are we going to really say is experimental and what is not, I think it is very, very difficult and very costly for any of the communities, especially rural communities, to be handling this isolated.

These are the things that we need in addition to financing mechanisms for rural communities; and I believe that we will be able to handle all Americans through integrated delivery systems, including the medically uninsured, the Medicare population under risk contracts, and as we are demonstrating now the many, many, many Medicaid folks. I believe we also could deal with the immigration issue at a later time.

Senator DURENBERGER. A last question, if I may, Mr. Chairman.

Is there some reason why you all did not come in here and say every American should be able to come into the system through an accountable health plan? We should not have one level of access for the so-called medically assisted, another level for the working poor, a third one for the elderly and the disabled, a fourth one for small businesses, a fifth one for the big employers of big businesses and a sixth one for rural areas and urbans and so forth.

Why did not any of you come in here and just say the goal ought to be every American ought to be able to have the security of an accountable health plan? And for the low income, you know, we drop Medicaid and there is a low income subsidy for the elderly. You have to be able to get rid of their Part A, Part B. The movie actor buys a supplemental and so forth.

Why did you not come in and just sort of lay it on the line here, that we cannot come out of this without the legislation that identifies the accountable health plan?

Mr. DIETRICH. Senator, I think from our perspective one of the mistakes that will really cause a lot of harm, especially in the rural environment, if reform relegates the private employer's concern only to what they pay and to whom they pay it. And by that I mean, if we take the employers—and rural America is foundationed by employers—if we take the employers out of the ability to drive solutions within those communities that all they worry about is, I am going to pay X dollars per employee per month to an accountable health plan or to whatever, we have taken a lot of the real leadership out of these rural communities that is stepping forward to find solutions, not just for their employees and dependents, but for the community as a whole.

Because employers in rural America recognize that the overall viability of the community is critical to their being about to continue to do business.

Senator DURENBERGER. Are you saying employers should be integrating the systems?

Mr. DIETRICH. I am saying that the thing that scares me about some of the reform initiatives is that as an employer, especially when you start moving the ERISA exemptions levels to $5,000 and things of that nature, you have taken away a lot of the real leadership in rural America that is out there now trying to come to grips with solutions in partnership with medical providers.

The reform initiatives that we talked about earlier with malpractice and liability in those, there are another set of reforms out there that are going to thwart the process and those are many of the State initiatives—the any willing provider legislation, no gatekeepers and all that.

So there are solutions out there that are being developed every day. Our concern is that reform do not thwart those solutions by taking away from the private sector the ability to control its own destiny.

Senator DURENBERGER. But what most of you see out there, what is happening—and I do not want to call it an accountable health plan, except that is what I happen to call it—I mean, you are seeing integration of the various services, whether they are insurance or hospitals or whatnot. That is happening out there.

If you could just give it a name and avoid having it show up the same way in Arkansas that it does in Mississippi or Minnesota or Montana, I am going to call it an accountable health plan.

You know, that is the vehicle for change. The employer does have a role. We have a role. But the vehicle for change is the concept of the accountable health plan.

Mr. DIETRICH. If the accountable health plan is a true partnership between the payers and providers within a piece of geography where together they are coming together and assuming the financial risk, then we will be okay.

But our fear is that in this process many of the employers are going to be relegated to a secondary position. I think we will use a lot of our leadership in rural America if that happens.

Senator DURENBERGER. Well, that is our problem.

Mr. BUSCH. Senator Durenberger?

Senator DURENBERGER. Yes.

Mr. BUSCH. From the Montana perspective, or at least from our perspective in Culbertson, one of the strengths of the MAF model is the flexibility it provides and the involvement it allows a community to design a health care provider model that will work for that community.

Senator Baucus mentioned that some of the openings that you have been at, you have been surprised at the number of people that come to it, almost more than are in the town itself. I think that reflects community involvement in the process and it is designed, I think, individually as a ground floor set of regulations. But beyond that an MAF can develop according to what the community requires.

Also, in a truly rural facility or area the MAF of the small rural hospital is one of the primary employers in that community. That and the school system are really the base around which the community survives. The rural health facility locally is essential also to recruit new business. Many businesses will not come into a town if there is not health care service there.

Certainly in rural areas agriculture is one of our largest business areas. It is a high risk occupation. Without emergency room services, it puts the population at risk.

But within all that similarity there is a tremendous amount of uniqueness. I think that flexibility within the plans is essential. I also wanted to mention very quickly that my experience has been with the MAF that it has really encouraged the development of this gatekeeper model. We provide a great deal of primary care service—preventive, diagnostic and then referral; and also we are involved in telecommunications which enables us to contact other facilities.

Dr. HARTMANN. I would like, if I could, to just add that I think there are a couple of different ways to interpret your question. But separating the notion of the source of payment from how many providers there are, I think in general most of us probably feel there should continue to be a variety of providers who can be responsive to the needs of their populations.

But I do think the research does tend to show that a single payer type system is the most cost effective. It does not eliminate the multiple providers at all. It maintains that kind of diversity. But it does appear to create a lot of efficiencies, which has been supported by the Congressional Budget Office.

Senator DURENBERGER. We have one like that and it is called Medicare.

Dr. HARTMANN. Exactly.

Senator DURENBERGER. The more you do, the more you get paid. So when the prices are racheted down by people sitting around here, you just see twice as many—you know, do you do twice as many things to people? That is the side of the Canadian system that we need to learn something from.

Dr. HARTMANN. Right.

Senator DURENBERGER. You have complemented them on the other side, which is good, but not on the single payer side.

The CHAIRMAN. Thank you, Senator Durenberger.

Senator Baucus?

Senator BAUCUS. Thank you very much, Mr. Chairman.

I must compliment Mr. Busch on his comments. He answered one of the questions I was going to ask, that is the flexibility. Walter, could you go on a little more and just give people even a more detailed flavor of the importance of that flexibility, say Culbertson compared with other rural communities, not only in Montana, but in other parts of the States, and the need for that flexibility in order to get the kind of participation and enthusiasm as you have described.

Mr. BUSCH. As you know better than I, each town in Montana has its own unique history and there is a great deal of civic pride in what goes on in the town. Some MAFs have only a mid-level practitioner available. Ours and one other have a physician and a mid-level practitioner or two. Some are relatively close to a secondary level facility, others are very far apart.

The MAF regulations as written enable each community to respond to the realities around their town.

Senator BAUCUS. Now, are there other alternative role models that perhaps are less flexible that might be a bit concerned with, and if so, what might they be?

Mr. BUSCH. The other one that I am aware of is that each RPCH model—that is another project being experimented with in seven States—I had a peripheral knowledge of that. What I have seen in that is that it requires a linkage of a small facility to a larger facility, 75 beds or larger, which would put us out of circulation right there. We are not near any bed——

Senator BAUCUS. Just tell everybody how far is it from Culbertson say to Billings, which is probably the major hospital that is closest to it.

Mr. BUSCH. Three hundred miles.

Senator BAUCUS. So you would have to drive 300 miles to get it?

Mr. BUSCH. For tertiary care.

Senator BAUCUS. For tertiary care.

Mr. BUSCH. As you know, our winters, we are dealing at 40 to 60 below temperatures with ground blizzards. So even going 20 miles can be a very hazardous experience in midwinter in Montana.

Telemedicine has helped a great deal. We were able to communicate directly with Billings, with the patient and our physician.

The CHAIRMAN. And you will soon have TeleVision.

Mr. BUSCH. Yes, sir.

Senator BAUCUS. Yes, sir.

Mr. BUSCH. We are part of a demonstration project initially funded by U.S. West and now by the OAA.

Senator BAUCUS. So you have fiberoptics? Do you have fiberoptics?

Mr. BUSCH. This is compressed digital. We are probably going to convert to fiberoptics. Rural cooperatives have purchased the U.S. contract, so I think we will be converting.

But we have been able to assist in some really important diagnoses over the television with the patient in bad weather in Culbertson, talking to the specialist in Billings. But distance is a tremendous.

As I listened to the testimony, you have talked definitions. One of the definitions that probably needs to be addressed is rural. What do we mean by rural?

You know, Kingston is rural in New York, but it probably would be considered urban in Montana.

Senator BAUCUS. I appreciate your saying that because that is so true. I mean, I am astounded by the sense of abrafobia of people from the east that they have when they come to Montana and other States west of the hundredth meridian where it does not rain. Where it does not rain there just are not very many people.

I remember when the First Lady was in Montana in April of last year for a health care hearing, I mean she understood it. That is, the difference between western rural and eastern rural, just immediately, instinctively, intuitively, when she said, this is not rural. This is mega rural. This is hyper rural. I mean it is true.

People from the east—and I just say this factually—who have spent not much time in the west just do not have an appreciation of how rural rural is in Western United States, that is in the northern high plain States and that part of the country. The distances are just phenomenal.

This is an anecdote, for whatever it is worth. I remember Senator Gorton, Slade Gorton from Washington, told me years ago he and his family bicycled across the country. They started in Seattle and they went across the country and ended up on the East Coast. He said he realized how big Montana was when he calculated, I think, about a quarter of the time across country was in Montana. I mean, it was not quite that, but that was the impression, the sense that he had.

The CHAIRMAN. Well, I can say that in the high school textbooks of this country in the year 1900, most of that part of America was just labeled "Great American Desert."

Senator BAUCUS. We are fighting that, because there are some Rutgers professors that want to return it to the Buffalo Commons, too.

The CHAIRMAN. They like it that way.

Senator BAUCUS. Right.

One other point though, do you think it is—how important is it to people in communities like Culbertson and Circle, Montana, for example, that the MAF concept be made permanent in statutory language? Is that important?

Mr. BUSCH. I think that the model become permanent is essential to the well being of the communities, both from the standpoint of health and from the standpoint of the economy. I do not believe that we would survive under the traditional model.

Under each RPCH model, I think we would have a difficult time surviving. We are not linked directly or close to any hospital at 75 beds or more, number one. And number two, as I see that each RPCH will understand it, it encourages that the small facility become pretty much a feeder facility to the larger facility. I believe if that happened, we would gradually lose enough volume that we probably could not be viable, plus we would probably lose a number of our health professionals who would not like that model.

So I think the MAF, I hope that can be made permanent. I think it has worked extremely well and I think your help has been a tremendous benefit to Montana. I hope that can be extended around the country.

Senator BAUCUS. Well, thank you.

Thank you very much.

Mr. BUSCH. Thank you, sir.

The CHAIRMAN. If I could just ask Mr. Ullmann, you probably do like the satellite arrangements?

Mr. ULLMANN. Yes, I do.

The CHAIRMAN. Because among other things, distances are not that great.

Mr. ULLMANN. Yes. One other thing we have done for rural America because we realize our database will never be large enough to really produce outcomes. So we have gone into joint ventures with the largest HMOs across the country and we have also entered into electronic transfer of technology with larger institutions and also get our research now on the experimental procedures and the latest drug technology from larger companies.

So if we can get that in rural America, that database will be richer.

The CHAIRMAN. Right. Well, I note, and I do not know if you are aware of this, but you and CoreSource are competing at Fort Edward. I see that you are back at Fort Edward now. I hope you are getting along reasonably well. [Laughter.]

The French and the English did not get along very well at Fort Edward, if you have seen the Last of the Mohicans.

There is a little land bridge about seven miles between Fort Edward on the Hudson and Fort George on Lake George, which if you can cross that land bridge you can paddle a canoe from New York Harbor to Montreal or to Quebec. That is why there were all the great battles such as Saratoga which took place there 12 years later. That was during the great war for the continent. If it were not for that, we would all be speaking French.

For what it is worth, it was in 1918 that the United States first required a non-United States citizen to have a passport entering this country. That is how recently this is. We think of it as an enormous burden.

I want to thank this panel so very much. We are very aware that there are three or four areas of rural activity. I mean, I think the area that you represent, Mr. Ullmann, it is not agricultural. Some. You are moving over into Delaware County where we live, which is sort of agricultural. But there are probably only 40 dairy farms left. These are urban populations that live in the countryside.

Whereas, you, sir, represent people who still really are rural and agricultural. Agriculture is their principle activity. Not all of them, but in Arkansas that is the sort of people you have. It is probably much the same in parts of Mississippi.

Then you have a situation such as you represent, Mr. Busch, which is not properly described as rural. These are the Great Plains and distances are vast. It is not fair to call it desert. But when you get past the hundredth meridian and it stops raining, it is not unfair to call the place desert.

We have to think about all three of them because it is a big country. We thank you very much for your very informative testimony. There will be some questions Senator Grassley suggested. We hope that you can respond so that they will be in the printed record.

With that our hearing is concluded.

[Whereupon, at 12:40 p.m., the hearing was concluded.]

APPENDIX

PREPARED STATEMENT OF STANLEY HOYT BLOCK, MD

Mr. Chairman and members of the committee, the National Association of Community Health Centers (NACHC) is the national membership organization of over 700 community, migrant and homeless health centers providing comprehensive primary care services to over 7 million medically underserved Americans in 1400 sites across the country.

NACHC and its member health centers are well aware of the failures of our health care system, in particular because we care for millions of Americans who have been forgotten or left behind—unserved, or poorly served at best—by the existing health care system. In this context, **health centers strongly support the President's call for meaningful health care reform to provide universal coverage to all Americans that can't be taken away, and improve access to care—especially to preventive and primary care, and contain health care costs.**

The needs of the underserved in health care reform are clear, and attainable this session of Congress:

The underserved need a place to go for entry into the health system—*a medical "home" that responds to their unique needs,* that is geographically and physically accessible, culturally and linguistically competent, and available during evening and weekend periods; and that offers comprehensive primary care and "enabling" services, like transportation, translation and outreach. Universal coverage, though essential, is not enough, as health insurance alone will not necessarily guarantee access to needed health care services;

The underserved need an adequate supply of *physicians and health professionals* who are trained to understand and respond to their unique needs and health care problems; and—

They need *the assurance of knowing that the essential community providers which have historically served them will be able to continue doing so,* through initiatives that provide adequate reimbursement (taking into account the inherently higher costs of caring for them) and risk contracting safeguards designed to protect their fiscal solvency.

Clearly, we now have the best opportunity in over half a century to extend access to affordable, quality health care to every American. **We want to work with the President and Congress to capitalize on this golden opportunity—let's make health care reform work for all Americans.** Many items of apparent consensus in Congress on health reform would make vital contributions toward improving access to health care and ensuring health security by:

- extending comprehensive coverage to millions of people who are currently uninsured or inadequately insured, with benefits equal to or better than those offered by many of the largest companies;
- eliminating the most brutal current health insurance industry practices of denying or discontinuing private insurance coverage because of previous or current health conditions, or due to a change or loss of job;
- proposing to substantially reorient our health care system—including the training of physicians and other providers—to focus more on low-cost, high-payoff preventive and primary care, including coverage of important preventive services;
- proposing to expand and improve preventive and primary health services in underserved rural and inner-city areas;

- recognizing and safeguarding the key role of health centers and other "essential community providers" in caring for low income and underserved communities.

With the inclusion of these elements, national health reform can lay a solid foundation for ensuring that every American—no matter what their circumstances—has access to affordable, quality health care.

However, with the notable exception of the single-payer plan, many of the major proposals for health care reform—particularly the "managed competition" approaches, which have received so much attention of late—contain elements that raise concerns about how well or poorly the system will meet the needs of the underserved. The proposals, most notably the Health Security Act and the Managed Competition Act sponsored by Representative Jim Cooper, rely heavily on a system of managed competition, under which several health plans—most of the managed care type—will compete for enrollees, ostensibly on the basis of price and quality of care. This focus on managed competition could work to assure care and at the same time contain costs for most Americans. Yet while managed care has been cited frequently for its successes in effectively organizing available local health resources to hold down the cost of care, there is no evidence that the presence of managed care in a community has successfully *increased* the level of available resources there, a critical factor in improving the health of underserved communities.

Moreover, *most managed care entities and HMOs have historically avoided the underserved because of their unique needs and inherently higher costs.* In a market-based, competitive health system with a foundation in managed care, the most expensive patients the underserved and those in greatest need of health care—could encounter significant discrimination and barriers to obtaining health care services. For some areas and populations—in particular low income, rural and inner-city minorities, and other at-risk Americans—this approach may not improve access to care, and could even prove detrimental. Because of factors such as geographic isolation, poverty, homelessness, and occupational hazards (not to mention the social-environmental threats that permeate low income/underserved communities), the underserved are at higher risk for serious and costly health conditions (accidents, high-risk pregnancies, child health problems, AIDS) than the general population. Thus, **organized delivery systems will have every incentive to avoid enrolling and serving them.** The provision of insurance coverage to the underserved is not an assurance that organized delivery systems will seek to provide quality services to these populations. What is absolutely clear to us is that a safety net will still be needed in a reformed system under a managed competition approach—a "front door" into the health care system that is significantly influenced by the medically underserved themselves.

Our concerns are further heightened by the limited nature of proposed federal cost-sharing assistance for low income persons and families in the various proposals for health reform. In this respect, the President's plan is among the most generous; other bills have severe limits. Nearly all bills would limit subsidies to the premium charges by plans that are at or below the weighted-average premium. *This limitation could effectively restrict the choice of poor persons to only low cost plans. thus running the risk of creating a de facto two-tier system.* Similarly, even the poorest Americans will face some cost sharing, including copayments for doctor visits and prescription changes. This burden will have its most telling effect on pregnant and postpartum women, infants, and those with chronic or complicated illnesses, because they will need frequent care and multiple medications.

Some of the many potentially serious problems that could be faced by low income Americans and the working poor in a managed competition-based system include—

- *Severely Restricted Choice of Plans or Providers:* Because of the restricted subsidies under the managed competition proposals, individuals with family incomes below 150% of the Federal poverty level are unlikely to be able to afford the premium surcharges for higher-cost plans. By this standard, 60 million people—25% of the entire population—will be able to choose only among the lowest-cost plans, and will be subject to the discrimination and poor quality often associated with the Medicaid program. It is unclear whether or to what extent low-income and other medically vulnerable populations will be assisted to enroll in plans, select a plan that works best for them, and to obtain the care and services they need, which in many cases go beyond the care and services included in the required package and furnished by traditional plans.
- *Lack of Plan Capacity:* Those who can afford only a low-cost plan may find there are not enough such plans available with enough capacity. Few plans will be willing to market coverage at the premium charged by low-cost plans, and will instead target employer-insured families.
- *Increased Discrimination and "Redlining":* If the new system is inadequately financed, health plans will have every incentive to avoid areas with high num-

bers of low-income people. Fly-by-night or "lowball" plans may well be the only providers bidding for coverage in these low income-areas—resulting in diminished access and lower quality services for *all* enrollees there. Depending on how Alliance and plan service areas are delineated, major redlining could occur, with low-income, racial/ethnic minority, and high-risk populations gerrymandered into segregated Alliance and plan service areas and subject to less oversight and poor quality care. Given the practices of managed care entities in Medicaid, private health plans are also likely to red-line traditional providers of care to underserved communities, thereby excluding entire high-risk neighborhoods. This red-lining is already happening as the health system across the country organizes itself for reform. The experience with redlining under Federal voting rights and credit lending laws suggests that no duty not to redline can counteract wide discretion in drawing and operating in identifiable service areas.

- *Obstacles to Specialty Care:* Lower-cost plans are more likely to require stricter utilization review and place more obstacles between low-income patients and specialty care. In particular, persons with chronic illnesses or disabilities may be adversely affected if plans are permitted to severely restrict out-of-plan referrals or payment for specialized care and services. Also, plans will presumably be required to cover out-of-area services (at least for emergency/urgent care needs). However, it is not clear yet how this will work under most of the major plans. This is a critically important issue for migrant farm workers, transportation employees and others whose work requires frequent and extensive travel, and involves multiple employers.
- *Inadequate Monitoring of Quality and Access:* Based on the experience with Medicaid, states and Alliances may not be able to adequately monitor quality and access in low-cost plans, especially when faced with the pressing need to hold down the cost of care.

Simply put, underserved Americans are in the health care predicament they are in because they have been rejected by the private market. The health center programs were enacted by the Federal Government in response to the failure of market forces to meet the needs of underserved and vulnerable populations. Thus, if market forces work for health care like they have worked in other sectors of the economy, underserved people and communities run the risk of being red-lined, short-changed and, in the end, getting far less care than they need or deserve.

Finally, undocumented persons are ineligible for coverage under virtually all major proposals, and are barred from receiving public subsidies or employer-subsidized benefits under the managed competition approaches (thus disqualifying millions from the employer coverage they now have). All hospitals presumably would still be required to furnish emergency care to undocumented persons under Federal anti-dumping law, but potentially hundreds of millions—if not billions—of dollars in uncompensated care would remain, with as yet no clearly identified funding source to cover the cost.

These concerns underscore the critical need for a substantial, Federally-administered "safety net" for millions of disadvantaged and underserved Americans, even after reform is implemented. Several major reform bills acknowledge this principle, but their response falls seriously short on some key elements. For example:

Access to Care: The Health Security Act's Access Initiative calls for a vital investment of about $4.5 billion over 6 years in the expansion of primary care services in underserved areas, in assisting in the formation of service delivery networks, and in furnishing key 'enabling services,' such as transportation and translation services, to those living there. Similar efforts are proposed in many of the other bills, as well. We strongly support the basic purpose of this Initiative and believe that the levels proposed by the President are minimally adequate to meet the need for such efforts (greater efforts are called for in the single-payer bill, at $4.8 billion over 6 years, and in the Chafee bill, at $5.6 billion over 5 years). However, nearly all of the President's funds would be administered under a *totally new, discretionary program,* which would give greatest preference to entities, including non-publicly assisted HMOs, private doctors and other institutions, with little or no community involvement or accountability; publicly-funded providers who band together are given a lower preference for receiving support.

What's more, we see it as a vote of no-confidence on the ability of disadvantaged and minority communities to positively influence the structure and character of their community's health care system. In our view, this represents a significant change of heart by the Administration on its early guarantees that health reform would help empower medically underserved communities.

Further, the discretionary nature of this new program (which is also found in other health reform proposals, with the exception of H.R. 1200) raises the distinct possibility that existing programs, such as the health centers, Family Planning, MCH, and Ryan White, which will continue to fill vitally important purposes even after reform is implemented, will be pitted against proposed new programs for scarce federal resources. Senators Fritz Hollings and Tom Harkin have fought as hard or harder than most other Members of this institution for funding for these programs, yet have been unable to keep their funding on par with general inflation, much less health inflation. A discretionary funding construct for a health reform access initiative raises the distinct probability that funding levels for these programs will never be adequate. The Managed Competition Act contains exceedingly limited resources, none of which could be used to expand capacity in underserved areas. The Senate and House Republican bills do contain resources for this purpose, but as put forth, could not be used for the formation of community-based networks and plans. Only the single-payer bill guarantees funding for these purposes. Given what is at stake, we feel that mandatory funding is the only viable approach.

Essential Community Providers: We applaud the Health Security Act and the Ways and Means Health Subcommittee bill for their unique and vital provisions that would recognize those who currently care for the underserved (such as Federally Qualified health centers and rural health clinics) as "essential community providers" (ECPs), and extend certain rights, such as contracting and payment requirements. These protections are found in only one other legislative proposal—that of Senator Chafee, where they would apply only to providers serving the Medicaid population, or about 15% of all eligible Americans.

Required contracting is the most appropriate way to assure an equitable sharing of responsibility for caring for high-risk populations, and to avoid red-lining and discriminatory practices. Adequate payment rates for essential providers will ensure that the health status of higher risk patients will not be adversely affected by managed care enrollment. At present, no system or methodology exists to adequately risk-adjust capitated payments to account for risk differentials among enrolled patients. Until an effective risk-adjustment methodology is developed and implemented, those providers who disproportionately serve high-risk individuals, if placed at excessive financial risk, could face financial ruin or be forced to skimp on necessary care in order to survive. On the other hand, because they serve disproportionate numbers of high-risk patients, adequately compensating health centers for their care can serve to make risk levels more reasonable for other providers. Medicare HMOs receive risk-adjusted payments in accordance with Sections 1833 and 1876 of the Social Security Act. Requiring reasonable-cost based payment to essential providers would offer nothing more to them than Medicare HMOs are already receiving—essentially, it requires the health plan to "pass through" the mandated risk-adjusted payment to the essential provider caring for the highest-risk populations. The last thing policymakers want to see happen in health reform is an erosion of health care infrastructure in underserved areas.

Under the President's bill, all health plans are required to contract with ECPs in their service area. ECPs that elect to contract on an "in-plan" basis (most health centers are likely to do this) will be paid no less than other providers for the same services by the Plan. ECPs that contract on an "out-of-plan" basis (most likely, school-based clinics, health care for the homeless, etc.) will be paid based on the Alliance-developed fee schedule or the most closely applicable Medicare methodology (for a health center, FQHC cost-based reimbursement), at the ECP's choice.

While these safeguards are critically important, we fear they do not offer adequate protections for ECPs. Most importantly, ECPs get precious few safeguards from *risk-based contracting* by health plans. Risk adjustments and reinsurance are required *only* for the health plans; there are no provisions requiring that they be shared with contracting providers—not even the ECPs who, more than any other, will face the inherently higher costs of caring for sicker and harder-to-serve patients. A possible scenario, even with the Health Security Act's safeguards: a health plan agrees to contract with the ECP, but on a risk basis; the health plan assigns the ECP the sickest patients, and pays the ECP no less—but no more—than other providers for the same services, with the ECP at risk for any costs in excess of the health plan's capitated payment. The ECP is out of business in 2–3 years.

NACHC believes that one overriding policy should govern the construct of an Essential Community Provider initiative: *those providing comprehensive primary care services to the underserved should be paid an adequate rate. and should be exposed to minimal risk.* Ensuring the continued function of essential providers will be absolutely critical if we are to encourage more caregivers to provide primary care, especially where it is most needed, and ensure that more of the underserved receive primary care and preventive services. From the viewpoint of health centers, the Ways and Means Health Subcommittee's Essential Provider amendment is the strongest such proposal offered thus far in the health reform debate.

Health Professions Education and Placement: Most of the major reform bills call for substantial reform of the nation's health professions education and training efforts, and restructures its financing. However, it leaves the lion's share of the resources in the hands of the nation's medical schools and teaching hospitals—which have played no small role in the current oversupply of specialists and our critical shortage of primary care physicians.

None of the legislative proposals effectively involve health centers in the training and education of health professionals. *Community health centers affiliated with teaching programs* have produced hundreds of family physicians, general internists and general pediatricians—exactly the kinds of doctors our health system desperately needs—yet they *get nothing in the way of direct funding to continue or expand their educational efforts.* Currently health centers with teaching programs are required to affiliate with a sponsoring medical school or teaching hospital. Payment for the costs of the health center's educational program is made on a "pass-through" basis with the sponsoring institution. The result is that many "teaching health centers" end up eating a substantial portion of the costs of their educational efforts. Further, the availability of residency opportunities in health centers is directly linked to the availability of teaching hospitals willing to engage in educational partnerships with them.

Health centers would like to have direct access to medical education funds so we can provide practice opportunities for medical residents and expose more medical students to the benefits of providing primary care in an underserved area. The available literature shows that where medical residents and other health professions students are exposed to primary care training in a community-based setting, significant numbers enter primary care as a practice. For the reformed health system to function successfully, it will have to generate significant numbers of new primary caregivers. Community and migrant health centers anxiously await the opportunity to participate in those professionals' education.

MAKING HEALTH REFORM WORK FOR UNDERSERVED AMERICANS

We believe that, **if health reform is to work for underserved Americans, it must empower medically underserved communities to develop workable, permanent, responsive community health care systems,** through steps to provide:

a substantial investment of guaranteed resources for the formation of community-based, consumer-directed health plans and networks, and to increase access to primary and preventive care in underserved areas, through support for key programs that now support vital services to disadvantaged and underserved populations (including the health center programs, Family Planning, and others).

strengthened safeguards for Essential Community Providers that assure preservation of the existing safety net in underserved communities, and their full participation in the new health care system, including safeguards against excessive risk in contracting with health plans and payment of rates that acknowledge the inherently higher costs of serving underserved populations;

direct funding for community-based training programs for primary care health professionals in order to assure adequate primary care educational opportunities for students in the most appropriate settings—where they are needed most.

NACHC has developed perfecting amendments to the various health reform proposals to meet these critical objectives.

The most pressing need of—and the most rational response to—the medically underserved under any health care reform approach is increased availability of community-responsive, consumer-directed, comprehensive primary health care services, particularly under a market-driven approach to reform where the bottom line will take absolute precedence. Yet more can and should be done than just investing in service development: *the lesson of the health center programs is that, although it may not be possible to empower communities to take control of the entire new health system, it is possible to empower them to own and operate their own entry points into it.* Health centers were founded with a vision of community and consumer empowerment, and their experience over the past 30 years provides an object lesson on how consumer involvement and community empowerment can succeed where other models have failed. *In this sense, health centers may be the last. best hope for communities in shaping their health care system and making it responsive to their needs.* For obvious reasons, we strongly believe that any access initiative worthy of the name should retain and significantly expand upon the health center model because:

- it is a proven model of getting Federal funds to improve the health of hard-to-reach populations to the areas that need them most;
- health centers represent a multibillion dollar investment by the Federal government in primary care infrastructure in underserved communities over the last 30 years, and attracting and retaining health professionals in shortage areas;
- have proven their effectiveness, cost efficiency and quality, and success in;
- it is a proven model of empowering underserved communities to manage their own points of access into the health system, and to tailor the services provided by the center to the unique needs of the community;
- the centers are accountable for efficient utilization of Federal funds and quality of services provided, and are subject to strict monitoring and oversight by Federal agencies, unparalleled in the private sector.

Policymakers should look hard at what has worked and why. and what has not worked for the underserved:

- Who has provided culturally competent care and ACCESS to these communities? Who has not?
- Who has seen all regardless of the ability to pay? Who has not?
- Who has kept costs in check while developing innovative approaches to meeting the health needs of these communities? Who has not?
- Who has attracted, trained and kept physicians and qualified health professionals in underserved communities? Who has not?
- Who has genuinely empowered communities to develop long-range solutions to their health care needs? Who has not?

Members of Congress can and must make sure that health care reform "stays on track" and works for our communities. Congress knows what works and should renew its commitment to Community Health Care. *This is not about a program, but rather an approach to empower communities to develop and direct long range solutions that will work for them*—in keeping with the President's principle of responsibility, which we all support.

In summary:

- President Clinton made a commitment to equality of access to health care. We fully support that pledge, and believe that health reform must work for all Americans, and especially for the medically underserved.
- There is much to admire and support in the President's proposed plan and those of other Members; at the same time, some elements cause considerable concern about how well these plans will address the most pressing needs of underserved Americans.
- Health care costs will never be controlled unless high-risk, underserved populations have access to primary and preventive care. Health insurance while essential, will not alone guarantee access to needed health services.
- Health reform should build on what has worked: the health center programs. Nothing else has our uniquely successful, 30-year track record of controlling costs, providing access to quality care, retaining health professionals where they're most needed, or empowering communities to develop long-range solutions to their health needs. Health reform should invest in such successes.
- We are committed to support and work with the President and the Congress to ensure the earliest possible passage and enactment of an effective, comprehensive national health reform plan this year.

Thank you.

PREPARED STATEMENT OF WALTER S. BUSCH

In a 1990 report in the Journal of Rural Health, Drs. Hart, Ammundson and Rosenblatt stated that

"rural hospitals play a unique role within the spectrum of hospital services in the United States. Rural Hospitals, although they are much smaller than their urban counterparts—are not merely scaled down versions of their city cousins. The common denominator of small rural hospitals is that they make available a menu of basic services to their local communities . . . the evidence shows that rural hospitals continue to concentrate on the basic "plain vanilla" services which are within the competence of local healthcare providers . . . these hospitals are basic public service organizations, for the most part community owned and community run, more akin to public wishes than entrepreneurial ventures."[1]

Regarding the financial impact of rural facilities on the National Healthcare budget, the authors go on to state that

"although rural hospitals appear to play an important role in the provision of basic health services to local populations that are often distant from alternative sources of care, the national fiscal impact is smaller. In fact (if they closed) it is quite probable that aggregate costs would rise, rural patients with relatively low-intensity medical needs were displaced to much more capital intensive and expensive urban hospitals, even if the increased transportation costs are not considered."[2]

*Source: Is There a Role For The Small Rural Hospital? Ammundson, Hart, Rosenblatt, WAMI, 1989.

FLEXIBILITY

Rural Healthcare facilities are important to their communities for many reasons, including access to primary and emergency care, financial stability (generally one of the largest employers) and perhaps most importantly, because they represent an important part of the fabric which binds together the many aspects of rural community life. While intangible, this is a reality well worth preserving.

I believe one of the great advantages of the MAF demonstration is precisely that it addresses this reality, and is designed with enough flexibility to allow the model to fit itself to the needs and capabilities of the various frontier communities where it is in service. Although it certainly is structured to require networking with larger facilities located in distant towns, it does not force one to one linkages which effectively would lead to loss of local autonomy of healthcare services. The MAF establishes a "floor," or minimum set of standards which must be met, but does not set a ceiling, so that each MAF develops along similar but yet unique lines, according to the needs of the respective communities and the service capabilities of the MAF.

I consider it to be a brilliantly conceived model which enables the full potential of each facility to be realized, and yet does give this within well established monitoring safeguards.

The Inspector Generals report on the MAF Demonstration (copy attached) issued in 1993, was highly complimentary of the quality of the services provided, and the cost effective manner in which this was being accomplished.

MAF: LOW IMPLEMENTATION COST, HIGH LEVEL OF ACCEPTANCE

Perhaps the best indication of its positive qualities is the support it has received among Montana facilities. Since 1990, six sites have been certified, and a seventh is in the application process. This has been accomplished without any HCFA grant support to those rural facilities, and only $100,000 per year to the program coordination site. (Montana Hospital Research and Education Foundation directed by Keith McCarty). This is a dramatic contrast to the $200,000.00 grant awards that are given to the RPCH sites to evaluate and implement a coordination effort with the EACH facilities.

By comparison, the MAF Demonstration has expended only $500,000 dollars to date with six sites operational, the EACH-RPCH has expended or is committed to spend approximately 17 million with less facility participation at this point in time.

I believe that the MAF program has worked even without large grant awards because of the inherent attractiveness of the program to frontier facilities and communities: it preserves local community control, it is simple to operate, and it has a proved track record. I believe this same experience would occur in any frontier area in the United States where the MAF was a choice.

ROOSEVELT MEMORIAL MEDICAL CENTER

One Example of an MAF Conversion

Roosevelt Memorial is a community owned, not-for-profit acute and long term care facility, partially supported through tax levies. The town of Culbertson was incorporated in 1887, and its first doctor arrived in 1901, followed by a hospital in 1902. Culbertson has had continuous hospital service since that time, with the present facility opened in 1977.

Roosevelt Memorial currently serves a population of approximately 2000 people, with about 900 residing within the city limits. Other towns in our healthcare district are Froid (15 miles North), Ft. Kipp (7 miles West), and Bainville (15 miles East). The geographic area within the district is over 380 square miles.

It was during a period of community wide economic distress that the facility began to reevaluate its healthcare mission in terms of what the community needed and would support, and what the facility could afford to provide in a high quality manner.

The Board of Trustees requested support from the WAMI Program (Washington, Alaska, Montana, Idaho Rural Health Project under the University of Washington), and AHEC (Area Health Education Center), under Dr. Frank Newman, to develop a meaningful strategic plan based upon community input and financial reality.

The evolutionary process towards primary care had begun. It is very important to note that the process, though assisted by experts outside the community, was from the start a community directed effort led by a locally elected and appointed Board of Directors.

As a direct result of this strategic planning effort, RMMC requested approval from the State of Montana to be licensed as a Medical Assistance Facility, and requested a Medicare Waiver from HCFA. Both were ultimately granted and Roosevelt Memorial became a functional MAF in December of 1992.

MAF: Local Service/Area Wide Networking

Our MAF, a ten bed acute care facility, then became the hub around which the various primary care services offered at RMMC were unified.

Specific changes in this strategic conversion to a primary care, integrated health service model included closing the obstetrical and surgical suites, while simultaneously developing a broad spectrum of outreach services needed by the community and within the capability of the facility, including a Certified Rural Health Clinic, a Certified Home Health Agency, a WIC Program, and a Community Wheelchair Accessible Van Service. In-patient acute and long term care, as well as 24 hr ER coverage, continued basically as before, but with a 96 hour admission limit and other MAF specific protocols.

Further, networking with other medical facilities and health agencies was incorporated into the MAF model, and includes contractual arrangements for such specialty services as Radiology, Pathology, Nutrition and Social Services, Physical and Occupational Therapy, Mobile Ultra-sound and Mammography, Child and Adult Immunization, Speech Therapy, Foot Care and Health Education with four providers (three secondary and one tertiary level). Under the EACH-RPCH model, linkage with one specific facility would seriously reduce the potential for optimizing supportive services which is possible as an MAF through selection among several providers, each with different areas of strength and expertise, and each with a co-equal relationship to the MAF.

It is important to note that the MAF is not likely to generate sufficient revenues as a stand alone, limited service acute care facility to cover its operational expenses. However, by its very presence it has a synergistic effect on other healthcare services, since it is the vehicle which attracts physicians and physician extenders as well as other healthcare professionals to the area. A direct relationship between long term care services and the provision of acute care services in rural areas is also essential for this healthcare delivery model to be successful.

Grants: Transition, Telemedicine

Roosevelt Memorial has benefited from several federal grants which has enabled it to convert many of its dreams to reality, including a Department of Transportation Grant which assisted in the purchase of our 14 passenger wheelchair accessible van, and a Rural Health Transition Grant, which helped in the recruitment of a second physician assistant to implement a new GYN service and share in the primary care rotation, as well as providing funds to build a garage to house our ambulance on site, and to train the ambulance volunteers to the level of Emergency Medical Technician.

Roosevelt Memorial is also one of six sites selected to participate in a US West Demonstration project to evaluate digitally compressed telemedicine capabilities (and subsequently funded for three additional years by a Rural Electric Association Grant).

Roosevelt Memorial is the only MAF participant in this grant, and we have found that the technology can play a very important role in providing quality healthcare services at the local community level. We have arranged specialist consultations between Board Certified Dermatologists, Radiologists, Pediatricians, Pulmonologists and Cardiologists located in Billings (300 miles away), and patients at Roosevelt Memorial, with their local physician or physician assistant also participating in the consultation. The success of this concept can be measured not only in terms of improved access to specialty care, but also in the added credibility it has provided to RMMC in the view of its patients, who can now come to our facility for care and yet be seen by specialists located in Billings, Miles City, Glendive or Sidney, Montana.

Other networking has developed among ten area hospitals and nursing homes through participation in the Montana Health Network, which was begun in 1986 as a health consortium among facilities in central and eastern Montana, and one tertiary center in Billings, to address the unique challenges or rural healthcare delivery. Among programs developed and implemented by this group are Trustee seminars, RN recruiting, health insurance, Workman's Comp., Quality Improvement and efforts to develop a Family Practice Residency Program in Montana.

EFFECTS OF THE MAF ON ROOSEVELT MEMORIAL

The discussion of Roosevelt Memorials experience is intended to illustrate the multi-faceted approach to healthcare services which is made possible through the Medical Assistance Facility Demonstration Project.

Without the MAF opportunity, local access to healthcare services would have been dramatically reduced or even ended. instead, as a direct-result of our participation in the MAF project, our financial status has stabilized and we have been able to recruit one full time family physician and one additional physician assistant. Our medical staff is now comprised of one supervising physician and two physician assistants, each of whom share call to assure coverage 24 hours per day, 7 days per week. I have attached some specific data about the MAF program to this paper, but would like to note two MAF components which have been especially important to us:

(1) Expanded use of physician extenders: they can admit to the MAF, accept call, and cover the emergency room without the supervising physician being in close proximity. We have provided training support for them to become Certified in ACLS (Advanced Cardiac Life Support) and PALS (Pediatric Advanced Life Support) and to participate in the Advanced Trauma Life Support Programs.

(2) Cost based reimbursement: under this reimbursement methodology, HCFA reimburses MAF's for in-patient acute care days based upon Medicare allowable costs, rather than DRG's (prospective payment). For low volume, high Medicare utilization facilities, this results in financial stability not otherwise possible.

CONCLUSION

The Medical Assistance Facility has improved access to quality health care services in a cost effective manner. It has restored healthcare services to four remote, rural communities, and prevented loss of service in two others. The program has cost relatively little to implement, and has been well received by both residents and rural communities. It is a very flexible program, and yet one that has provided consistently high quality care.

Based on my personal experience in the MAF program, I strongly recommend to the Committee that consideration be given to expanding the MAF model to the National level.

I would like to thank Senator Baucus for inviting me participate in this hearing, and Senator Moynihan and members of the Finance Committee for including my testimony in your schedule.

Also, the very existence of the MAF Demonstration is in large part the result of the interest and support provided by Senator Baucus and his staff over the past five years, and on behalf of all the MAF facilities and the people served by them, I extend my sincere gratitude.

The day to day support has been provided by Jim Ahrens of the Hospital Association and Keith McCarty of the Montana Hospital Research and Education Foundation, in addition Sheldon Weisgrau, Project Officer of the Health Care Financing Administration, has been very helpful with concerns regarding the Demonstration.

Department of Health and Human Services
OFFICE OF
INSPECTOR GENERAL

MEDICAL ASSISTANCE FACILITIES

A DEMONSTRATION PROGRAM TO PROVIDE ACCESS TO HEALTH CARE IN FRONTIER COMMUNITIES

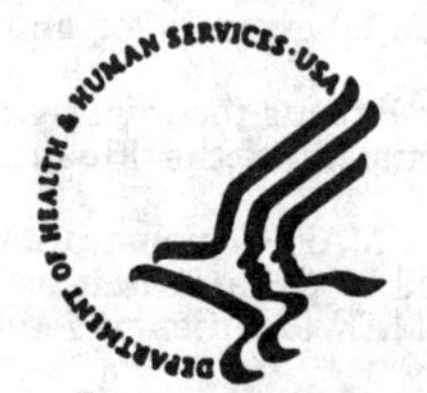

JULY 1993   OEI-04-92-00731

EXECUTIVE SUMMARY

PURPOSE

To describe the Health Care Financing Administration's Medical Assistance Facility demonstration program and its effect on access to inpatient health care in frontier Montana.

BACKGROUND

Concerned that hospitals closing in frontier Montana left residents without access to basic health care, the Montana State legislature authorized a Medical Assistance Facility (MAF) program in 1987. The program was designed to provide continued access to health care by converting a full-service hospital into a low-intensity, short-stay health care service center. Montana law allows MAFs to provide up to 96 hours of inpatient care. MAFs must be located more than 35 road miles from the nearest hospital or be located in a county with a population density of no more than 6 residents per square mile.

Montana revised its licensure rules to reduce hospital staffing requirements and adapted other existing standards to the MAF concept. MAFs are allowed to offer any health service for which it is adequately equipped and staffed to perform.

Montana's MAF program received a Health Care Financing Administration (HCFA) demonstration grant to fund planning and program development activities. Also, HCFA authorized a waiver of over forty hospital Conditions of Participation so that MAFs could receive Medicare reimbursement under Medicare Part A on a cost basis. Current HCFA waivers and grant for the MAF program are scheduled to end in 1993.

SCOPE AND METHODOLOGY

In December of 1992, we visited and reviewed MAF operations at each of four Montana communities that had converted formerly closed hospitals into a MAF. The MAFs are located in Circle, Jordan, Terry and Ekalaka. We also reviewed relevant State and Federal legislation, regulations, service records, and other appropriate documentation. We interviewed program officials in Montana, HCFA, and each of the four Montana communities.

FINDINGS

HCFA's MAF demonstration program provides access to inpatient care in frontier areas without a hospital

MAFs provide up to 96 hours - or 4 days - of limited inpatient services in four frontier Montana communities. The average length of stay is 2.4 days.

MAFs also provide inpatient care primarily to elderly members of the communities -- 72 percent of MAF patients are over 65 years of age.

Finally, MAFs provide 24-hour emergency health care services and outpatient care to the four communities.

MAFs facilitate a health care network in frontier areas

MAFs attract other service providers to the facility. For example, each MAF offers dental services once a week. Special care providers such as physical therapists and mobile mammography units use the MAF as a center to offer care to the community.

MAFs also serve as a hub for a referral network, referring patients to hospitals for advanced care, nursing homes and home health services.

Flexibility in staffing is critical to success of MAFs

Non-physicians, such as a physician assistant, admit patients and provide medical care in MAFs. They do so under the supervision of a physician who can be in a different town. Each MAF provides service within the skill level of its employed medical professionals. Also, when a MAF has no patients, it may close. The flexibility allowed in MAFs help attract and retain medical professionals in frontier areas.

MAFs appear to be cost efficient

For these four frontier communities, MAFs appear to be cost efficient due to more efficient use of staff and less operating cost when compared to a small underused frontier hospital. Further, MAFs may be located closer to patients, which encourages cost efficient preventive health care and reduces patient transportation cost.

CONCLUSION

MAFs hold promise as a viable alternative for frontier community health care. The MAF program is a practical and flexible way to provide access to basic inpatient and emergency medical care in frontier areas -- particularly those that are struggling to keep a failing hospital open, and those that do not have adequate local health care. The results of this review and HCFA's upcoming formal evaluation can be used jointly by HCFA in determining whether to (1) continue the MAF concept in Montana, and (2) apply it in additional frontier communities.

MEDICAL ASSISTANCE FACILITIES

A MONTANA MODEL
FOR RURAL HEALTH CARE FACILITIES

OVERVIEW

MEDICAL ASSISTANCE FACILITY

A) <u>Project Objective</u>

    1.   To demonstrate that the MAF option can prevent the permanent loss of health care services resulting from hospital closure

    2.   To demonstrate that patients will accept the MAF as an alternative to full service hospitals

    3.   To demonstrate that the MAF provides high quality health care services at no greater cost to HCFA than a full service hospital

    4.   To demonstrate the MAF option as a model for implementation in other states

B) <u>Services Provided</u>

    1.   In-patient care for up to 96 hours

    2.   In-patient care prior to transport to a secondary or tertiary hospital

C) <u>Geographic Eligibility Criteria</u>

    1.   County with fewer than 6 residents per square mile

        and/or

    2.   Distance of more than 35 road miles from next present hospital

D) <u>Reasons for MAF Conversion</u>

    1.   Improved utilization of physician extenders (physician assistants, nurse practitioners)

    2.   Provider flexibility

    3.   Operational restructuring

    4.   Restoration or maintenance of access (see addendum)

    5.   Cost based reimbursement

    6.   Integration of services

E) <u>Health Care Services Through MAF Sites</u>

    1.   Local offering of preventative, primary, and acute care

    2.   Access provided to care not available in MAF
- Removal to other providers and facilities
- Contracted services
- Transfer agreements

    3.   Coordinated system of transportation for emergency and non-emergency cases

    4.   Community health focus

COMPARISON OF MEDICAL ASSISTANCE FACILITY (MAF) AND RURAL PRIMARY CARE HOSPITAL (RPCH)

	<u>Medical Assistance Facility</u>	<u>Rural Primary Care Hospital</u>
Geographic Limitation	Must be located in a county with fewer than six residents per square mile, or located more than 35 road miles from the nearest hospital.	Must be located in a rural area or in an urban county whose geographic area is substantially larger than the average area for urban counties and whose hospital service area is similar to the service area of hospitals located in rural areas.
Size Limitation	None	Not more than 6 inpatient or 12 inpatient beds if participating in the swing-bed program.
Length of Stay Limitation	96 hours (4 days) (Exceptions due to snow, flood, bridge repair or any circumstances beyond the control of the MAF are noted in the patient's record.)	72 hours (3 days) (Exceptions granted for inclement weather or other emergency conditions.)
Scope of Services	Mandatory services: - Inpatient medical care limited to 96 hours; - Emergency medical care; - Laboratory; - Pharmacy	Mandatory services: - Inpatient medical care for up to 72 hours; - Emergency medical care; - Laboratory - Radiology
Emergency Medical Services	Must be available and staffed on a 24-hour a day basis; minimum staffing is by emergency medical technician; registered nurses are on call and available within 20 minutes and medical staff members are on call and available within one hour from the time the patient first contacts the facility.	Must be "made available" on a 24-hour a day basis; staff with emergency care training or experience on call and available on site within 30 minutes.

Hours of Operation	24 hours/day when occupied by inpatients; when not occupied, ER is staffed 24 hours/day, 7 days/week by at least an EMT; RNs and physicians/NPPs on call.	24 hour/day when occupied by inpatients; when not occupied, emergency services must be "made available."
Admitting Criteria	PRO certifies medical necessity of all admissions.	A physician certifies that inpatient services were required to be furnished on an immediate and temporary basis.
Referral Relationships	Written agreements required with: - Hospital(s) - "Specialized" diagnostic imaging and laboratory providers; - Skilled nursing facility; - Home health agency; - Licensed ambulance service; - PRO or its equivalent.	Written agreements required with an Essential Access Community Hospital (EACH) for referrals, joint staff privileges, and data and communication systems.
Governing Board	Governing body is legally responsible for the facility and: - Appoints and supervises the medical staff; - Appoints chief executive officer; - Prepares and adopts institutional plans.	Governing body or responsible individual is fully responsible for determining, implementing, and monitoring policies governing the RPCH's total operation and for ensuring quality and safety of services.
Medical Staff	Composed of at least one physician and may also include one or more physician assistants and/or nurse practitioners; on call and available within one hour from the time the patient first contacts the facility.	Composed of at least one physician and may also include one or more physician assistants and/or nurse practitioners; on call and available on site within 30 minutes.

Nursing Staff	A registered nurse must be on duty at least 8 hours per day and be on call and available within 20 minutes at all times whenever there is an inpatient in the facility; a registered nurse must assign the nursing care of patients to other nursing personnel in accordance with the patients' needs and the qualifications and competence of the nursing staff available.	A registered nurse, clinical nurse specialist, or licensed practical nurse is on duty whenever the RPCH has one or more inpatients; a registered nurse must provide or assign to other nursing personnel the nursing care of each patient.
Quality Assurance	Governing body assures that facility has an effective, on-going, facility-wide, written QA program and implementation plan in effect that ensures and evaluates the quality of patient care provided; PRO concurrent review between 48th and 72nd hour of patient stay.	The RPCH has an effective quality assurance program to evaluate the quality and appropriateness of the diagnosis and treatment furnished and of the treatment outcomes.
Medicare Reimbursement	Facility-wide cost-based reimbursement, excluding distinct-part units.	Part A: Per diem for the first year; year-one per diem increased by PPS update factor for subsequent years; plan for prospective payment system for RPCH inpatient services. Part B: Facility may elect one of two methods: 1) a cost-based facility service fee with reasonable charges for professional services billed separately, and 2) an all-inclusive rate combining both professional and facility services combonents; plan for prospective payment system for RPCH inpatient services.
Grants	Cooperative agreement (approximately $100,000/year since June 1988) to Montana Hospital Research and Education Foundation; no grants to facilities.	Grants to seven states and participating facilities to support conversion to RPCHs, EACHs, and RHNs ($17.1 million awarded through 1993).
Authority	Waiver from Secretary (1990); state legislation (1987).	Federal legislation (1989); Code of Federal Regulations (1993); state legislation in some states.
Extent of program	1 state; 6 facilities (approximately 15 percent of eligible hospitals); 1 additional site in process.	7 states; 44 RPCHs and 31 EACHs.

Taken from LEARNING FROM THE MAF AND EACH/RPCH EXPERIMENTS: OPTIONS FOR A NATIONAL PROGRAM FOR RURAL HOSPITALS, George Wright, Anthony Wellever, Suzanne Felt, March 21, 1994.

GRANT SUPPORT
(in millions)

	EACH/RPCH		MAF	
	Number Participants	Amount Awarded	Number Participants	Amount Awarded
States	7	$3.7	1	$0.5
Support Hospitals	31	5.5	NA	NA
Limited Service Hospitals	44	7.8	56	-
Total		17.1		0.5

DEVELOPMENT OF THE MAF PROJECT

- ✔ 1986 - TASK FORCE RECOMMENDATION
- ✔ 1987 - STATE STATUTE CATEGORY OF LICENSURE
- ✔ 1988 - DEVELOPMENT OF MODEL
- ✔ 1990 - FEDERAL AUTHORIZATION
- ✔ 1990 - FIRST MAF IN MONTANA

MAF MEDICARE AUTHORIZATION

- ◆ **OBRA 1990**
  - **RURAL HOSPITAL DEMONSTRATION PROJECT**
  - **LIMITED SERVICE RURAL HOSPITALS**
  - **APPLICABLE TO ONLY MONTANA**
- ◆ **OBRA 1993**
  - **CONTINUATION OF MAF WAIVER TO JULY 1, 1997**

DOWNSIZING FROM HOSPITAL TO MAF

MAF Site	Hospital Beds	MAF Beds	LTC Beds	Swing Beds
Circle	20	2	18-No Change	1
Culbertson	14	10	44 - Added 4	4
Ekalaka	16	10	22 - Added 1	5
Jordan	12	2	18 - No Change	0
Terry	5	2	19 - Added 3	0
TOTALS	67	26	121 - Added 8	10

RESTORATION OR MAINTENANCE OF ACCESS

MAF Site	Loss of Access*	Restoration of Access**
Circle	6 months	December, 1990
Ekalaka	3 years	May, 1991
Jordan	5 years	August, 1991
Terry	6 months	January, 1992
Culbertson	No Loss	November, 1992

*　Time period that hospital portion of the facility was closed
**　Date facility was certified/operational to admit patients

TRANSFER AGREEMENTS

MAF Site	Primary/Seconday	Distance in Miles	Tertiary	Distance in Miles
Circle	Glendive Medical Center (Glendive)	44	Deaconess Medical Center; St. Vincent Hospital	242
Culbertson	Mercy Medical Center (Williston, ND)	44	Deaconess Medical Center; St. Vincent Hospital	310
Ekalaka	Fallon Medical Complex (Baker)	35	Deaconess Medical Center; St. Vincent Hospital	261
Jordan	Holy Rosary Hospital (Miles City)	85	Deaconess Medical Center; St. Vincent Hospital	175
Terry	Glendive Medical Center (Glendive)	35	Deaconess Medical Center; St. Vincent Hospital	184

CONTRACTED SERVICES AND CONSULTANTS

Medical Records	Speech Therapy
Dietary	Social Services
Physical Therapy	Pharmacy
Medical Staff	Utilization Review/PRO
Building Repair/Maintenance	Fire Safety
Pathologist	Ambulance
Bio-Med/Calibration	Psychology
Radiologist	Counseling
Financial/CPA	Home Health

MEDICAL STAFF COMPOSITION

MAF Site	On-Site	Practitioners	
		Medical Direction	Backup/Consultant/ Courtesy
Circle	MD, PA-C	Local	Yes
Culbertson	DO, PA-C	Local	Yes
Ekalaka	PA-C	Remote (35 miles)	Yes
Jordan	PA-C	Remote (85 miles)	Yes
Terry	PA-C	Remote (35 miles)	Yes

MAF INFORMATION RESOURCES

- **KEITH McCARTY**
  DIRECTOR, MAF DEMONSTRATION PROJECT
  MONTANA HOSPITAL ASSOCIATION
  1720 NINTH AVENUE
  HELENA, MONTANA 59604
  (406) 442-8802

- **DENZEL DAVIS**
  ADMINISTRATOR, HEALTH FACILITIES DIVISION
  MONTANA DEPARTMENT OF HEALTH
  COGSWELL BUILDING
  HELENA, MONTANA 59620
  (406) 444-2037

- **WALTER BUSCH**
  ADMINISTRATOR, ROOSVELT MEMORIAL MEDICAL
  CENTER
  P.O. BOX 419
  CULBERTSON, MONTANA 59218
  (406) 787-6281

- **FRANK NEWMAN**
  DIRECTOR, MONTANA OFFICE OF RURAL HEALTH
  MONTANA STATE UNIVERSITY
  BOZEMAN, MONTANA 59717
  (406) 994-6001

MAJOR DIFFERENCES BETWEEN HOSPITAL CONDITIONS OF PARTICIPATION AND MEDICAL ASSISTANCE FACILITY LICENSURE RULES

Hospital Conditions of Participation	MAF Licensure Rule
Every patient is under the care of a doctor of medicine or osteopathy; a doctor of dental surgery or dental medicine . . . ; a doctor of podiatric medicine . . . ; a doctor of optometry . . . ; a chiropractor.	Every patient is either under the care of a physician or under the care of a nurse practitioner (NP) or physician assistant (PA) supervised by a physician.
Patients are admitted to the hospital only on the recommendations of a licensed practitioner permitted by the State to admit patients to a hospital. If a patient is admitted by a practitioner not specified [above], the patient is under the care of a doctor of medicine or osteopathy.	Whenever a patient is admitted to the facility by a PA or a NP, the facility's sponsoring physician is notified of that fact, by phone or otherwise, within 24 hours after the admission. . . .
A doctor of medicine or osteopathy is on duty or on call at all times.	A physician, NP, or PA is on duty or on call and physically available at the facility within one hour at all times. . . .
The hospital must have an organized nursing service that provides 24-hour nursing service.	A medical assistance facility must have a nursing service that provides 24-hour nursing services whenever a patient is in the facility. . . .
The hospital must provide 24-hour nursing services furnished or supervised by a registered nurse and have a licensed practical nurse or registered nurse on duty at all times. . . .	A registered nurse must be on duty at least 8 hours per day, and the Director of Nursing or another registered nurse designated as the Director's alternate must be on call and available within 20 minutes at all times.
The hospital must maintain, or have available, diagnostic radiologic services.	If a medical assistance facility maintains, or has available, diagnostic radiologic services, they must meet the following standards. . . .
[The conditions of participation have no comparable standard.]	No patient is cared for in the facility for more than 96 hours.
[The conditions of participation have no comparable standard.]	The medical assistance facility must enter into agreements with one or more providers participating in Medicare or Medicaid to provide services meeting the needs of its patients which the facility itself is unable to meet.

From Abt Associates, Inc., *The Montana Medical Assistance Facility Demonstration Evaluation: Implementation Case Study* (draft), November 8, 1991, p. 6.

RESPONSES OF WALTER S. BUSCH TO QUESTIONS FROM SENATOR DOLE

Question: What are your principal concerns with the reform proposal you are hearing about? My principal concern is that the MAF Demonstration Project seems to be relegated to a one State option, even though the MAF is the only program of its kind with a successful track record. The EACH-RPCH model seems to be the program being given the most emphasis by HCFA, even though it is much more costly to implement than the MAF, and more likely to result in the closure of small rural facilities by their larger neighbors.

Question: Is further assistance needed?

Answer: Yes, the MAF Project does need assistance in two ways:

First, to become a permanent category of licensure within the Medicare program, and secondly, to be made available to qualifying remote, rural healthcare facilities in every state

Question: Are there other states/providers who are seeking to do what you have done?

Answer: Many states have expressed strong interest in the MAF program, and several (including Kentucky, Georgia and Florida) have passed provisions at the state level to implement models similar to the MAF Demonstration, but have been unable to obtain a Medicare Waiver from HCFA. The MAF program cannot function without a waiver, since Medicare patients would be excluded from reimbursement for services.

Question: Is there something we can do to assist them?

Answer: As mentioned previously, if the MAF received permanent designation within the Medicare program, then every state would be able to implement similar programs. This would be very helpful in maintaining essential access medical care in remote areas, and would serve to.improve the viability of the small community based.facility.

I believe that the MAF concept is far superior to the EACH-RPCH model for frontier medical facilities. I strongly encourage the Senate Finance Committee to consider making it available throughout the United States.

Thank you for your interest in the subject of Medical Assistance Facilities and rural healthcare, and for providing me with the opportunity to respond.

If I can be of any further assistance, please contact me. We have an excellent research office available in Montana through the Montana Hospital Research and Education Foundation, directed by Keith McCarty, and either he or I will do our best to provide whatever further information that may be required.

PREPARED STATEMENT OF JANE L. DELGADO

Members of the Committee, I am pleased to have this opportunity to offer the perspective of the National Coalition of Hispanic Health and Human Services Organizations (COSSMHO) on access to health care for Hispanic communities under health care reform. However, before providing our perspective on this issue I would like to provide you with some background on COSSMHO.

COSSMHO is the only national organization with a primary mission of improving the health and well-being of Hispanic communities. We represent the needs and concerns of over 350 community-based organizations and 1,000 professionals providing front-line health and human services in Hispanic communities. All COSSMHO programs utilize a community-based empowerment model of service delivery as evidenced by the fact that 60% of the COSSMHO budget funds community-based programs. COSSMHO also operates a computer bulletin board network of 350 Hispanic community-based organizations organized by 35 coordinating centers Founded in 1973, COSSMHO is celebrating its 20th anniversary as the nation's action forum for Hispanic health. Given our community-based health mission, COSSMHO does not accept funding from tobacco or alcohol companies or their subsidiaries, the only national Hispanic organization to have adopted this organizational policy.

Keeping with COSSMHO's community-based mission, our positions on health reform are based on a process that brought together a representative group of 68 Hispanic community health and human services leaders from across the nation, including the directors of community-based organizations, elected and appointed officials, city and county health officers, and academicians to assess and make recommendations for health care reform. The group met as a whole and after extensive deliberation developed a series of consensus proposals in three critical areas: (1) reducing the bureaucracy, (2) increasing revenue and cost containment, and (3) ensuring quality. Those proposals have formed a consistent Hispanic community message which has been provided to the White House and Congressional groups putting together health reform proposals, in a briefing to the President and Vice President, Congressional visits by COSSMHO membership and a series of Hispanic community town meetings on heath reform. That message can be summarized in three priorities:

(1) **Reduce the Bureaucracy Through True Universal Coverage.** Current proposals provide a different package of benefits to residents of Puerto Rico and do not provide a health card to undocumented workers. The exclusion of parts of a population who reside in a community is contrary to basic principles of public health. Moreover, it creates a costly and unnecessary bureaucracy to screen out persons not covered. Coverage of services must include mental health and preventive services on parity with other health services. Such services should be made available now rather than being phased in, which creates unnecessary administrative costs as new bureaucracies are set up with each new phase of services.

(2) **Generate New Revenue by increasing Taxes on Tobacco, Alcohol and Guns.** Providing a comprehensive universal system of health will require new revenue. The first sources of revenue used should be taxes on agents that drive up the costs of health care including a $2 per pack increase in the cigarette tax and increased taxes on alcohol, guns and ammunition. Such taxes are not only a source of new revenue but also help reduce future health costs by acting as a barrier to substance abuse and violence. In fact, it is estimated that raising the cigarette excise tax by $2 a pack would result in $23 billion in new revenue and save 1 million more lives than a 75¢ increase.

(3) **Ensure Quality Through Culturally and Linguistically Competent Systems.** Financial access to health care will not achieve a healthier nation unless quality services are provided. That includes providing culturally and linguistically competent services by linking them to reimbursement and licensing, ensuring access to community-based health and mental health providers, and including an Hispanic identifier on any universal claim form to determine if adequate quality services are being provided to Hispanic communities.

Today, 39.0% of the Hispanic community is uninsured compared to 24.0% of non-Hispanic blacks and 13.8% of non-Hispanic whites.[1] As the group most likely to be uninsured, Hispanics have a large stake in the enactment of health reform which meets the community's standards of a reduced bureaucracy through true universal coverage; new revenue from increased taxes on tobacco, alcohol and guns; and quality through culturally and linguistically competent systems.

I. REDUCE THE BUREAUCRACY THROUGH TRUE UNIVERSAL COVERAGE

The President's Health Security Act specifically excludes undocumented workers from health care coverage. Not covering undocumented workers will be an administrative and bureaucratic nightmare. Undocumented workers represent only about 1.6% of the nation's population.[2] Yet The President's health reform proposal seeks to screen every person for legal status when they enter the health care system. This process will divert funds from health care services to health care bureaucracy.

Coverage of all residents is in the public health interest. In order to protect the health of any particular resident of a community, you must cover all residents of that community. It is a basic principle of public health that not providing health services to a particular segment of a community puts the health of the entire community at risk. For example, in the measles outbreak of 1990, Hispanic children were 7.3 times more likely to contract measles than were non-Hispanic white children with a total of 13,323 measles cases being reported among the nation's preschool children.[3] In 1993 there were only 104 measles cases reported.[4] If a policy had been in place in 1990 not to provide immunization services to a specific segment of the pre-school age population, it is unlikely that in 1993 we would be witnessing a much reduced incidence of measles among children. Simply stated, disease and illness does not ask to see a "green card." The sound pubic health policy is to live up to the true meaning of universal coverage and provide services to all members of the community.

Undocumented workers pay $7.0 billion annually in taxes. What we know about undocumented workers and their use of public services does not square with the "public burden" arguments for excluding undocumented from health care services. Estimates of the costs of public benefits to undocumented workers have been overstated. The net public cost of undocumented workers in 1992 amounted to $1.9 billion or only $475 in public benefits per undocumented person.[5] One of the most widely used figures of the public costs of undocumented workers was calculated by Dr. Donald Huddle who estimated the net costs at about $11.9 billion.[6] However, there were a number of flaws in his calculation including using elderly populations in his estimate of AFDC recipients, assuming in his projection of the new immigrant population that no immigrants die or leave the country after 1992, and using a population figure for undocumented persons higher than that of the U.S. Census Bureau.[7] New figures, correcting for the Huddle study flaws, calculated by Dr. Jeffrey Passel of the Urban Institute and the Tomas Rivera Center found that the actual public costs for undocumented workers was about $8.9 billion in 1992 and that undocumented workers paid $7.0 billion in taxes (income, Social Security, sales, gasoline, etc.) The costs of public benefits to undocumented workers ($8.9 billion) minus the amount of taxes they pay ($7.0 billion) results in a net cost to government of $1.9 billion. While we hear much about the public costs of undocumented workers we rarely hear data on the other side of the equation—taxes paid by undocumented workers.

Only 4% of hospital visits by undocumented workers were paid for as "free care." Specific to health care services, the U.S. Department of Justice found in 1986 that in the 12 months before legalized aliens became legal, only 4% of those who had a hospital stay received uncompensated hospital care.[8] In addition, the study found that of those who entered the hospital for a pregnancy only 5% received uncompensated hospital care.[9] These figures are counter to much of the rhetoric about undocumented workers abusing the health care system. In fact, the Department of Justice study found that of hospital visits by their study group of undocumented workers, 47% of hospital visits were paid for by private insurance and 45% were paid for by the patient or the patient's family.[10]

The first tenet of public health is that any health care system must serve everyone in a community in order to protect the health and well being of that community. When a building is burning, firefighters do not ask first if the persons trapped in the building are legal residents. They put out the fire and save the people.

Not providing the same level of care to residents of Puerto Rico creates a two-tier health system. which negatively impacts on Puerto Rico and all the states in which Puerto Ricans reside The President's health plan would not provide the plan's full benefit package to residents of the Commonwealth of Puerto Rico. This proposal would leave a population of 3.5 million American citizens without the same access to care that the President would offer every other American citizen. Creating such a two-tier health plan is bad public health policy.

Mental health benefits are a critical Part of a comprehensive package. One of the most significant unmet needs of the Hispanic community is mental health benefits and the toll on the health and well being of the community is dramatic. For example, 12.0% of Hispanic high school students report making at least one suicide attempt compared to 6.5% of their non-Hispanic black and 7.9% of their non-Hispanic white peers.[11] A factor in this dramatic incidence of suicide attempts is a lack of access to mental health services in the Hispanic community. Overall, the rate of use inpatient psychiatric services by Hispanics (451.1/100,000 persons) is less than that of non-Hispanic blacks (931.8) and non-Hispanic whites (550.0).[12] Furthermore, a study of services in Los Angeles found that of persons with a recent DlS/DSM-III disorder diagnosed, Mexican Americans made half as many visits (11.1) to a mental health professional as did non-Hispanic whites (21.7).[13] For the Hispanic community, access to mental health services is a critical component of a comprehensive and quality health care system.

II. GENERATE NEW REVENUE BY INCREASING TAXES ON TOBACCO, ALCOHOL AND GUNS

There are precious few occasions when a legislative action will have such a clear and positive impact as will a $2 a pack cigarette tax increase. The $2 a pack cigarette tax increase would generate $23 billion in new revenue and each additional 25 cents of taxation beyond the President's proposed 75 cent increase will save approximately 200,000 lives with the $2 tax saving one million more lives than the 75¢ increase.[14] COSSMHO endorses the $2 a pack tax increase because it is progressive in terms of community health, it will create a significant barrier to initiation of smoking among Hispanic youth, and it will generate revenue to finance part of the public health burden created by smoking.

Cigarette tax is a progressive tax in terms of health. The tobacco industry has generated an uproar over the proposed tobacco tax increase contending that it is a regressive tax that will finance health care on the backs of the poorest Americans. That argument is offensive coming from an industry that has marketed disease to the communities least able to afford its consequences.

The tobacco tax is progressive in terms of community health because it will reduce smoking incidence and save lives. The Centers for Disease Control estimate that smoking now kills an estimated 435,000 persons every year in the United States.[15] In fact, smoking kills more persons in the United States annually than alcohol, heroin, crack, automobile and airplane accidents, homicides, suicides and AIDS combined.[16] Furthermore, environmental tobacco smoke—smoke from other people's cigarettes—has been identified as the nation's third leading cause of preventable death, causing approximately 35,000 to 40,000 deaths annually from cardiovascular disease among nonsmokers and 3,000 lung cancer deaths.[17] Environmental tobacco smoke is of special concern in Hispanic communities because of new research which demonstrates that of children ever exposed to smoke, Hispanic pre-school children while being the group least likely to be exposed to smoke prenatally they were the racial/ethnic group most likely to be exposed postnatally in the home.78

Cigarette tax will prevent smoking among youth. A $2 increase in the cigarette excise tax will prevent smoking initiation among youth. Currently 8.7% of Hispanic youth 12–17 years of age report smoking cigarettes in the past month compared to 4.3% of their non-Hispanic black and 12.7% of non-Hispanic white peers. Furthermore, 7.4% of Hispanic high school students report smoking cigarettes on 25 or more of the last 30 days to being surveyed.[19] Of particular concern is the fact that smoking appears to be increasing among Hispanic youth, particularly Hispanic women.[20] At the same time that smoking is increasing among Hispanic youth, tobacco companies have spent twice as much as any other industry on billboard advertising in Hispanic communities.[21] Billboard advertising is where preteens most often see cigarette advertising.[22]

A $2 a pack level of taxation would reduce the number of people who smoke by over 7.5 million and would prevent roughly 2 million premature tobacco-caused deaths over time.[23] The effect would be particularly evident among youth who are more sensitive to price than adults are in choosing to ,smoke. One study has estimated that the price elasticity of demand (price sensitivity) for cigarettes among teenagers is more than three times the elasticity figure for adults.[24] Given that half of all smokers start smoking regularly before 18 years of age,[25] the barrier to smoking initiation among youth is perhaps the most positive and long-lasting effect of a $2 a pack cigarette tax.

Cigarette tax will generate revenue. While the greatest benefits of the cigarette tax are the public health benefits of decreasing smoking and preventing smoking initiation, particularly among youth, the cigarette tax will also generate revenue to offset the health cost caused by smoking. The Office of Technology Assessment has estimated that each pack of cigarettes sold results in health care costs and lost productivity amounting to $2.59 per pack.[26] In 1990 dollars, it is estimated that smoking results in $501 billion in excess lifetime health costs for current and former smokers.[27] The cost grows by approximately $9–10 billion annually due to the additional excess lifetime health care costs of the one million teenagers who take up smoking each year.28

Federal, state and local governments collected about $11 billion in cigarette excise taxes in 1991.[29] Raising the cigarette tax by $2 a pack would generate approximately $23 billion annually in revenue.[30] Furthermore, this tax should be broadened to include all tobacco products, particularly snuff and chewing tobacco, use of which is increasing among high school students.[31] The tobacco tax increase is sound health policy both in public health benefits and fiscal benefits. A broad tobacco tax increase will decrease smoking; prevent smoking initiation, particularly among youth and generate revenue to pay for the health consequences of smoking. It is a progressive public policy which deserves to be enacted with dispatch.

Hispanic communities support tobacco tax increase. Perhaps the best proof that a tobacco tax is a progressive public policy is the support it enjoys in the Hispanic community. A recent poll of Californians demonstrated Hispanic community support for an increase in the tobacco tax. The poll found that a majority (51.4%) of Hispanics supported an increase tax on tobacco products compared to 46.3% of non-Hispanics.[32] Among current smokers, Hispanic smokers were approximately twice as likely as non-Hispanic smokers (37% and 19% respectively) to support an increase on tobacco products.[33] Furthermore, three-quarters (76.8%) of Hispanics compared to 54.4% of non-Hispanics supported a ban on tobacco product advertising on billboards.[34]

Given the public and community health benefits of the $2 tobacco tax and its potential for health care revenue development, the time has come to stop talking about reform and act on the first and easiest step to health care reform, the $2 tobacco tax.

An increased alcohol tax would counter an increasing trend of alcohol use among Hispanic youth. As in tobacco use, there is a sensitivity to price in the use of alcohol, particularly among youth. Increasing the federal excise tax on tobacco would be an effective method for preventing alcohol abuse among Hispanic youth. This is of particular concern since young Hispanic adults age 18–25 are more likely to be drinkers than older Hispanic adults over 45 years of age (53% compared to 27.8%).[35] Furthermore ,among youths age 12–17 years Hispanics are more likely to report alcohol use (23%) than their non-Hispanic white and black peers (both 20%).36

An increase in the federal excise tax on firearms and ammunition would support efforts to decrease the impact of guns on Hispanic communities. The mortality rate for homicide and legal intervention for Hispanic youth 15–24 years of age is 6.2 per 100,000 compared to 3.9 for their non-Hispanic white peers.[37] This mortality data details an increasingly violent environment Hispanic children are growing up in. In fact, a recent survey of parents found that 60.0% of Hispanic parents report that they "worry a lot" that their child will get shot compared to 6.0% of non-Hispanic white parents and 23.0% of non-Hispanic black parents who report the same fear.[38] An increase in the federal excise tax on firearms and ammunition would be a small step to help parents prevent the violence-in their children's lives due to guns.

III. ENSURE QUALITY THROUGH CULTURALLY AND LINGUISTICALLY COMPETENT SYSTEMS

Linking cultural and linguistic competency of care to reimbursement and licensing under heath care reform is critical to ensuring a quality system of care for Hispanic communities. A culturally and linguistically competent system of care is as important as scientific competency of the provider and financial access. The importance of culture in health care was recently demonstrated by a study which found that ethnicity of the patient was the most significant factor in obtaining quality health care services.[39]

A medical services study found that Hispanics were half as likely as non-Hispanic whites to receive adequate pain treatment. A recent study published in the Journal of the American Medical Association demonstrated the differential care provided to Hispanic patients and the need to make cultural and linguistic competency a primary concern for the health care system. The study conducted at the UCLA Emergency Medicine Center surveyed records of patients in 1990 and 1991 who entered the emergency room with an isolated long-bone fracture. Patients were excluded from the study if they had any complicating conditions other than the fracture or if the injury had occurred more than six hours prior to admission. For this specific medical condition, the researchers looked for a specific quality of care measure, administration of analgesia (pain medication). The results of the study were that Hispanics were half as likely as non-Hispanic whites to receive adequate treatment (administration of an analgesia).

These findings are significant because the study controlled for insurance status (all study patients had already gained admission to the emergency room), primary language, patient sex, provider characteristics, and time of presentation and time spent in emergency room. Controlling for these variables, the researchers found that Hispanic ethnicity was the strongest predictor of inadequate analgesia. This finding supports the importance of federally mandating cultural and linguistic competency of services as an essential standard to be assured by states through licensure and certification.

Inclusion of community-based health and mental health providers is vital for delivery of quality care to Hispanic communities. Community-based providers have traditionally provided care to underserved Hispanic communities. They have built a level of trust with their patients and the community and are a vital link to meeting the needs of traditionally underserved communities. A number of community-based providers, however, are private practice or small group physicians practicing in Hispanic communities and community-health centers which are not federally qualified. In fact, only 18.2% of federally qualified Community Health Centers serve a majority Hispanic client population compared to 71.7% of Migrant Health Centers which serve a majority Hispanic client population.[40] At the same time the FY'94 budget for Community Health Centers ($593.6 million) is more than ten times that for Migrant Health Centers ($58.01 million).

A number of community health centers providing services to Hispanic communities are not federally qualified because of regulations under section 330 of the Public Health Service Act that federally qualified health centers have a number of client population characteristics including a high infant mortality rate. In the Hispanic community infant mortality rates are similar to those for non-Hispanic whites (7.5 per 100,000 live births for Mexican Americans, 9.0 for Puerto Ricans, 5.9 for Cuban Americans compared to 7.1 for non-Hispanic whites and 17.5 for non-Hispanic blacks).[41] At the same time, however, Hispanic children exhibit high morbidity rates for preventable illness such as measles, active asthma, pediatric AIDS, school-days lost due to preventable illness and are the group of children to have the least number of pediatric visits.[42] Federal regulations recently recognized the importance of these morbidity indicators by adding them to the criteria for new federally qualified Community Health Centers.

The fact remains, however, that a number of community health centers currently providing care to underserved Hispanic communities are not federally qualified and will have to wait to make application when funds again become available under the new regulations which include morbidity measures in the definition of a federally qualified health center. Until such time, however, these providers must be included in any health reform plan. For this reason, language relating to delivering care to underserved communities should not focus on current federally qualified health centers but should instead focus on community-based providers who have a history of serving underserved populations.

Inclusion of an Hispanic identifier on a universal health claim form is vital to understanding the delivery of health services to Hispanic communities. Most health reform plans call for efforts to streamline the paperwork in health care. Currently, attention is centered on using Form HCHA–1450 [UB–82] and Form HCFA–1500 as the standard claim forms; neither of these forms includes an identifier for Hispanics or Hispanic subgroups. In order to understand the delivery of health care to Hispanic communities it is vital that any claim form include a racial/ethnic identifier. A move to a Standard claim form will mean that the vast majority of health services information will be based on information gathered through the universal claim form. Not including a racial/ethnic identifier on such a form would profoundly impede the ability of the health care community to understand the differential needs and service patterns of racial and ethnic communities. It would also significantly compromise the ability of fiscal planners to accurately predict and plan for the service needs of racial and ethnic communities in any managed plan of health services.

Thank you for the opportunity to present testimony before this committee. I would be happy to answer any questions.

[1] R. Valdez. "Insuring Latinos Against the Cost of Illness," Journal of the American Medical Association, Vol 269, No. 7.

[2] U.S. Census Bureau, Estimated Number and Percent Distribution of the Undocumented Population by State, 1993 and CP-1-1. Estimate of the undocumented population is 4,000,000 and total U.S. population estimate is 243,709,873.

[3] Centers for Disease Control and Prevention. "Measles United States 1990," Morbidity and Mortality Weekly Report, 40:369-372.

[4] Centers for Disease Control and Prevention. "Reported Vaccine Preventable Diseases," Morbidity and Mortality Weekly Report, 43(4):57-58.

[5] Jeffrey Passel, "Corrections in Estimates in 'Costs of Immigrants'" The Tomas Rivera Center, February 1994.

[6] Donald Huddle. "The Net Costs of Immigrants," in Passel.

[7] Jeffrey Passel, "Corrections in Estimates in 'Costs of Immigrants'" The Tomas Rivera Center, February 1994.

[8] U.S. Department of Justice, Immigration and Naturalization Service. "Immigration Reform and Control Act, Report on the Legalized Alien Population," March 1992.

[9] Ibid.

[10] Ibid.

[11] Centers for Disease Control. "Attempted Suicide Among High School Students--United States, 1990" Morbidity and Mortality Weekly Report, Youth Risk Behavior Surveillance System, Vol. 40, No. 37, September 20, 1991, Table 1.

[12] Lonnie R. Snowden. "Use of Inpatient Mental Health Services by Members of Ethnic Minority Groups," American Psychologist, March 1990.

[13] Richard Hough. "Utilization of Health and Mental Health Services by Los Angeles Mexican Americans and Non-Hispanic Whites," Archives of General Psychiatry, Vol. 44, August 1987.

[14] Coalition on Smoking or Health, "Saving Lives and Raising Revenue," January 1993.

[15] U.S. Department of Health and Human Services. "Reducing the Health Consequences of Smoking: 25 Years of Progress. A Report of the Surgeon General." DHHS Publication No. (CDC) 89-8411, 1989.

[16] Ibid.

[17] Council on Cardiopulmonary and Critical Care, American Heart Association, "Environmental Tobacco Smoke and Cardiovascular Disease," Circulation, August 1992, and U.S. Environmental Protection Agency, "Respiratory Health Effects of Passive Smoking," May 1992.

[18] National Center for Health Statistics. "Children's Exposure to Environmental Cigarette Smoke Before and After Birth." Advance Data, No. 202, June 18, 1991.

[19] Centers for Disease Control. "Tobacco Use Among High School Students--United States." Morbidity and Mortality Weekly Report. Vol. 40, No. 36, September 13, 1991.

[20] Escobedo, et. al. "Birth Cohort Analysis of Prevalence of Cigarette Smoking Among Hispanics in the United States," Journal of the American Medical Association, Jan. 6, 1989; Vol. 261, No. 1.

[21] Ronald M. Davis. "Current Trends in Cigarette Advertising and Marketing." New England Journal of Medicine. Vol. 316, No. 12, 1987.

[22] Gary Levin. "Poll: Camel ads effective with kids." Advertising Age, April 27, 1992.

[23] Coalition on Smoking or Health, "Saving Lives and Raising Revenue," January 1993.

[24] Lewit, et. al. "The Effects of Government Regulation on Teenage Smoking," Journal of Law and Economics. Vol. 24, December 1981.

[25] Centers for Disease Control. "Tobacco Use Among High School Students--United States." Morbidity and Mortality Weekly Report. Vol. 40, No. 36, September 13, 1991.

[26] Office of Technology Assessment, U.S. Congress. "Smoking Related Deaths and Financial Costs," September 1990 (Staff Memorandum).

[27] Thomas Hodgson. "Cigarette Smoking and Lifetime Medical Expenditures," The Milbank Quarterly, Vol. 70, No. 1, 1992.

[28] Ibid.

[29] The Tobacco Institute, "The Tax Burden on Tobacco," TI, Vol. 26, 1991.

[30] Coalition on Smoking or Health, "Saving Lives and Raising Revenue," January 1993.

[31] Centers for Disease Control. "Tobacco Use Among High School Students--United States." Morbidity and Mortality Weekly Report. Vol. 40, No. 36, September 13, 1991.

[32] Coalition on Smoking or Health, California Survey Report, 1993.

[33] Ibid.

[34] Ibid.

[35] U.S. Department of Health and Human Services. National Household Survey on Drug Abuse, Main Findings, 1991.

[36] Ibid.

[37] Centers for Disease Control and Prevention. "Vital Statistics of the United States, Vol. II, Mortality, Part A," 1950-1990.

[38] National Commission on Children. "Speaking of Kids: A National Survey of Children and Parents," Report of the National Opinion Research Project, 1991, Figure 21.

[39] Todd, et. al. "Ethnicity as a Risk Factor for Inadequate Emergency Department Analgesia," Journal of the American Medical Association, Vol. 269, No. 12, 1993.

[40] Health Resources and Services Administration. Special data run of community and migrant heath centers and ethnic composition of clients, 1993.

[41] National Center for Health Statistics. "Advance Report of Final Mortality Statistics, 1991," 42 (2) Supplement, August 1993.

[42] COSSMHO. "Growing Up Hispanic," Leadership Report, 1994.

RESPONSES OF DR. DELGADO TO A QUESTION FROM SENATOR PRYOR

Answer: In your testimony you discuss the need for health care providers who speak the language of the clients they serve.

In my home state of Arkansas,, I am proud to say that we are opening our very first health center for migrant farmworkers. Approximately 40,000 migrant farmworkers pass through the state of Arkansas every year, and between 7,000 and 8,000 have settled permanently in the Arkansas. Many of them work in the poultry industry.

My question is this: Many of our migrant farmworkers speak Spanish. The clinic administrator has had a difficult time locating Spanish speaking health professionals to staff this clinic. What recruitment advice would you have for this administrator, and for other clinic administrators who struggle with this same problem?

Answer: That migrant clinic director in Arkansas faces a difficult problem. Hispanics represent a small segment of those training for the health professions. According to the latest data from the Health Resources and Services Administration, while Hispanics represent approximately 9% of the U.S. population, they represent 5.4% of medical school students, 6.8% of dental school students, 4.0% of optometry school students, 4.2% of pharmacy school students, and only 3.0% of nursing school students. This is a small pool to recruit from in when seeking Hispanic health staff an even smaller pool in seeking Spanish-speaking Hispanic health professionals. While an intermediate step for that migrant clinic director may be to work with Hispanic health professional associations, her job will remain difficult until our training of health professionals reaches parity with Hispanic representation in the U.S. population. Clearly, there is a need in health reform legislation to target mentoring and scholarship resources to Hispanic health professional students and the institutions that train them.

Another part of the equation, however, must be to train all health professional students in cultural and linguistic competency. The U.S. Department of Health and Human Services has established a national goal for the nation under Healthy People 200'O to "increase to at least 50% the proportion of counties that have established culturally and linguistically appropriate community health promotion programs for racial and ethnic minority populations." In order to achieve that goal we must dramatically expand programs established under the Disadvantaged Minority Health and Improvement Act which focus on cultural and linguistic competency training of health professionals. In addition, I would recommend a look at Tufts University Medical School which is offering in-depth training in cultural and linguistic competency to a group of its medical students which includes coursework in the area as well as clinical placements in organizations delivering services to underserved Hispanic communities. It is an example of what should be happening at all of our health professional schools.

PREPARED STATEMENT OF ORLO L. DIETRICH, JR.

Mr. Chairman and members of the Committee: Thank you for the opportunity to appear today at this important hearing.

My name is Orlo S. Dietrich, Jr. and I am Executive Vice-President of CoreSource, Inc. Our company is a national managed health care and information firm that develops and manages health care delivery systems in non-urban and rural areas. Today, our company is the largest manager of rural health care delivery systems in the nation with 175 networks in 29 states serving more than 300,000 people. CoreSource and a predecessor company, Burgett & Dietrich, of which I was President, have been developing rural health care delivery systems since 1985. CoreSource assists local employers, physicians, and hospitals in organizing community-based, primary care networks, and linking these networks into integrated health care delivery systems. The community-based, primary care networks localize health care spending and strengthen the viability of the local medical community.

As the Administration and Congress take up the complex task of health care reform legislation, I want to commend the Chairman and this Committee on the special attention being given to health care delivery in rural areas. As you know, there is justifiable concern that many of the proposals for reforming the health care delivery system are designed primarily for urban settings. Many rural areas have fragile health care provider communities as a result of: limited numbers of providers, disproportionate numbers of elderly, low-income, and uninsured individuals, and sparse populations. Many rural areas are unable to support multiple, competing health care networks. Nevertheless, as someone who has witnessed and worked for the growth of innovative health care delivery systems in rural areas, I know that national health care reform can work in rural areas.

The private sector can develop health care delivery systems that work on a localized basis in rural areas. Rural delivery systems can deliver comprehensive coverage to all rural residents. What is important is that national legislation take account of conditions peculiar to rural areas. National legislation must be flexible, recognizing that rural areas differ from urban areas and rural areas differ from each other.

Health care reform legislation should enhance opportunities for private-sector creation of local primary care networks, and linking networks to rural, integrated health care delivery systems capable of accepting various risk arrangements for fully-insured care. Above all, reform legislation should seek to strengthen and revitalize fragile, rural health care communities through health care plans that keep local as much care as possible and that reduce the referral of care to metropolitan centers. Medical dollars must be increasingly spent in the rural areas and less spent on specialists, facilities, and health care plans that are located in larger, but distant, urban areas.

In this testimony, I will first discuss how CoreSource facilitates the development and successful management of community-based, primary care networks, and then links these networks into rural, integrated health care delivery systems. Second, I shall describe how private-sector primary care networks and integrated health care delivery systems can meet the requirements that will be expected of health care plans under the major reform proposals. Third, I will make a few specific suggestions as to the unique features of rural health care delivery systems that may require special consideration in fashioning health care reform legislation. Fourth, I will discuss necessary modifications to the Medicare and Medicaid programs to encourage their beneficiaries' participation in rural primary care networks and integrated health care delivery systems.

I. DEVELOPMENT OF COMMUNITY-BASED, PRIMARY CARE NETWORKS AND INTEGRATED HEALTH CARE DELIVERY SYSTEMS

CoreSource focuses its business on small cities and towns and their surrounding rural areas. Traditional managed care programs have generally steered away from these smaller communities. Increasingly, over the past ten years, CoreSource has found that major employers in a non-urban area have had a strong interest in improving local health care delivery, while controlling costs. In recent years, CoreSource has also found increased commitment by local hospitals and physicians to sponsor the development of managed care, integrated delivery systems that serve local employers and residents. CoreSource assists these motivated sponsors to design and administer community-based, primary care networks. CoreSource combines these networks into risk-bearing, integrated health care delivery systems, which offer rural individuals and employers high quality and cost-effective health care programs.

CoreSource's experience in designing integrated health care delivery systems for rural areas suggests the importance of the following strategies:

- *Primary care networks.* A community-based, primary care network should be open to all qualified providers. Primary care physicians serve as care managers for their patients. The network must be highly selective in its referral of patients to tertiary care providers and hospitals in urban areas.
- *Managed care techniques.* The integrated health care delivery system should employ state-of-the-art managed care techniques, including a comprehensive information system that educates providers and facilitates effective utilization review.
- *Collaborative, integrated health care delivery system.* A community-based, integrated delivery system must involve full participation in management by providers, employers, and patients. The system must be large enough to support risk-bearing managed care programs.

CoreSource-designed integrated health care delivery systems succeed because they are community based. CoreSource systems are not local franchises of a national insurance plan or company. Each network is designed and governed locally. Financial sponsorship may be provided by a self-insuring employer, a group of employers, a local hospital, or groups of physicians. Risks and rewards related to cost containment are typically shared by community providers and employers. Medical dollars are kept in the local community, under local control. This community-based approach to managed care makes everyone responsible for and committed to a network's success.

CoreSource fosters collaboration by involving representatives of all parties in the governance and management of the primary care networks. Networks are managed by local, representative boards that continually evaluate health care objectives and provider performance. The community boards monitor consumer satisfaction and track the overall financial performance of the network. The collaborative, community-based approach to management encourages a willingness to cooperate in the enforcement of cost containment objectives and peer review and quality assessments.

The primary care physician is a patient's primary access point to the health care delivery system. Each patient chooses a primary care physician who serves as care manager and provides non-emergency care or a referral to specialists that are part of the network. All local primary care physicians who meet accepted credentialing standards are offered the opportunity to participate in the network. However, the network is more selective in its inclusion of specialists and hospitals, especially those outside of the local area. The network insists that specialists and hospitals adhere to stringent standards for quality care and cost-effective operation.

Cost containment is achieved primarily through state-of-the-art management of utilization of health care services. Sound utilization management depends on a sophisticated medical information system. CoreSource, through its extensive national experience, assists in developing an information base on patient outcomes, practice patterns, and local costs. Local, regional, and national performance indices are developed that serve as benchmarks for provider performance.

Primary care physicians are routinely provided information about their patient's care, regardless of who is providing the care. The primary care physician is then able to assess his or her own practice patterns, as well as the practice patterns of referral providers. The continual case management that is provided by a primary care physician enhances the overall quality of care, while also contributing to cost-effective operation of the network and the integrated delivery system.

CoreSource-designed networks seek full participation by willing local primary care physicians. Employees and rural residents choose voluntarily to join the network. Employers are attracted by the opportunity to control costs while assuring high quality care. Smaller employers and self-employed individuals can be drawn into the integrated delivery system. CoreSource links primary care networks to provide sufficient participants to support a community-based delivery system that can accept and manage risk.

CoreSource takes great pride in the results obtained by its primary care networks. Over the last decade, CoreSource networks have kept annual cost increases to single digit levels during periods when annual increases in indemnity insurance plans and in HMOs averaged well in double figures. All CoreSource networks, dating back nearly a decade, continue to operate today. These networks average 80-90 percent voluntary enrollment levels among eligible employees.

II. RURAL NETWORKS CAN MEET REQUIREMENTS FOR HEALTH CARE PLANS UNDER MAJOR REFORM PROPOSALS

A common objective of the major health care reform proposals is providing universal coverage. Under most of the major reform proposals, universal coverage would be facilitated by certain requirements imposed on health insurance and health care plans. These requirements relate to matters such as open access, area-wide availability, guaranteed renewability, no adverse selection, community rating, basic benefits packages with cost-sharing, standardization of claims and information reports, and quality assurance. We wish to stress that community-based, primary care networks and integrated health care delivery systems serving rural areas could meet these common requirements that would apply to other insurance plans and urban-centered networks. We believe that through integrated health care delivery systems and their community-based networks, individual residents of rural areas can be offered access to the same basic benefits package and be protected by the same insurance reform rules as urban and suburban residents.

We do not testify today as regards the specifications of a basic benefits package or insurance reforms. However, we wish to highlight those common features of health care reform proposals which rural health care delivery systems should be able to offer:

- *Open enrollment.* Rural health care delivery systems and their primary care networks could be established that would not exclude from coverage any eligible resident of the rural area.
- *Area-wide eligibility.* Rural health care delivery systems could be available throughout a designated rural area.
- *Guaranteed access and renewability.* Rural health care delivery systems could meet any requirements prohibiting the taking of medical histories or financial conditions into account in accepting residents for enrollment. Enrollees could be guaranteed renewability absent fraud or nonpayment of premiums.

- *No discrimination based on health status.* Rural health care delivery systems could meet requirements prohibiting limitations or exclusions of benefits relating to preexisting conditions, health status of enrollee or dependents, claims experience, receipt of health care, or lack of insurability.
- *Basic benefits package.* Rural health care delivery systems could offer all residents of rural areas a basic benefits plan, subject to prescribed cost-sharing.
- *Community rating.* Rural health care delivery systems could charge premiums based on community rating methodologies.
- *Information management.* Rural, integrated health care delivery systems and their community-based, primary care networks can participate fully in any national claims and information management program, including electronic information systems.
- *Ouality assurance.* Rural primary care networks could implement any required quality assurance program, including peer review and outcomes analysis.

It should be emphasized that certain of the above requirements, such as open access, area-wide eligibility, and guaranteed renewability are not generally provided today in either rural or urban markets. Making these features available will, everywhere, require some restructuring and redesign of health plans and provider networks. In rural areas, with their smaller populations and sometimes differing risk profiles, primary care networks may require special incentives, transition rules,.or other considerations before becoming fully established. In the next section of my testimony, I discuss some of these special circumstances of rural networks and integrated health care delivery systems and how they might be addressed in health care reform legislation.

III. SPECIAL CONSIDERATIONS OF RURAL AREAS AND COMMUNITY-BASED NETWORKS

We suggest that an overarching objective of rural health care provisions in any reform legislation should be ensuring that rural communities are served by local, community-based, primary care networks and integrated health care delivery systems. Small towns and rural areas should not be served only by extensions of urban-centered, managed care plans. Maintaining a viable delivery system in rural areas requires that care be directed from within, and out-of-area referrals be limited to circumstances in which the local medical providers can not serve area residents. CoreSource's success in designing integrated health care delivery systems and primary care networks that improve quality while controlling costs has been predicated upon keeping the medical dollars within the local community.

To support community-based, primary care networks and integrated health care delivery systems, Congress should encourage private-sector sponsorship of these systems in rural areas. A considerable investment of funds is needed to organize and establish primary care networks and integrated health care delivery systems. Beyond the start-up investment, any health care delivery system or plan must be established on a viable economic footing.

Our experience demonstrates that vigorous participation by. employers and providers is critical to development of successful and well-managed networks. When employers take responsibility for a substantial portion of their employees' health insurance coverage, employers have a powerful incentive to control costs without compromising quality. self-insured employers are often most familiar with taking direct responsibility for managing their employees' health insurance coverage. Based on our experience, health care reform legislation should not diminish the role of employers, including self-insuring employers, in managing their health care costs. Specifically, legislation should encourage employers, at least in rural areas, to actively participate in the financing, organization, and governance of rural primary care networks. For smaller employers who can not self-insure their employees' benefits, legislation should provide incentives for their participation in integrated health care delivery systems sponsored by others.

A second indispensable part of community-based, primary care networks and rural, integrated health care delivery systems is direct involvement of primary care providers and local hospitals in the organization and management of primary care networks. Because the supply of physicians is likely to remain too thin in most rural areas to support multiple competing health networks, physicians should be allowed to organize rural health care delivery networks. Physicians should actively participate in governance, and this implies a correlative right to share in the risks and rewards of the performance of the network. Local community hospitals, too, should be encouraged to sponsor or participate in rural, integrated health care delivery systems.

Some of the existing health care reform proposals envision a wholly arm's-length relationship between physicians, hospitals and health insurance companies or health plans. While this separation may make sense in urban markets that can support competition among multiple insurance companies and plan sponsors, in rural areas, a more flexible approach is called for. A further important reason to permit physicians and hospitals to have a financial stake in a rural, health care delivery system's success is the need to keep medical dollars in the rural community. One means of attracting and retaining rural physicians is to give them a financial interest in the success of managed care in the rural community.

Most of the current reform proposals also envision some type of solvency requirements being imposed upon health plans. Whatever solvency requirements may be authorized for large urban-centered plans, special considerations should be given to rural, integrated health care delivery systems and their community-based, primary care networks. Obviously, rural residents need to be protected from the risk of insolvent plans. The point we stress is that different solvency standards will need to be applied to rural health care plans.

The major health care reform proposals also envision some provision for so-called risk adjustments between plans in a state that have comparatively high- and low-risk populations. However the concept of risk adjustment is implemented for urban-centered plans, special considerations will be required for implementation in rural areas that support only one or two primary care networks or integrated health care delivery systems.

IV. PARTICIPATION BY MEDICAID AND MEDICARE BENEFICIARIES IN RURAL, INTEGRATED HEALTH CARE DELIVERY SYSTEMS

Health care reform legislation should address the special problems involved in the participation by Medicare and Medicaid beneficiaries in rural, integrated health care delivery systems. Current federal and state requirements under the Medicare and Medicaid programs present barriers to beneficiaries' participation in rural, integrated health care delivery systems. Certain rights provided to Medicare and Medicaid beneficiaries would, if applied to rural integrated delivery systems, impede the systems' ability to coordinate and improve the quality of care and impose unnecessary administrative costs.

For Medicaid beneficiaries, we suggest that a minimum eligibility period of six months be established for selection of a rural health care delivery system. Disenrollment should not be arbitrary, but only for good cause, with a predetermined re-enrollment period. Matching federal funds should be made available to encourage states with shorter eligibility periods to establish this minimum eligibility period.

Medicare and Medicaid beneficiary enrollment in rural, integrated health care delivery systems should be encouraged, by mandating the offering of these systems and fee-for-service options, by reimbursing rural networks for the higher administrative costs in expanding enrollment, and by educating beneficiaries about the newly available networks. Enrollment reporting and confidentiality requirements need to be made consistent with private sector requirements.

Further, the current "75% Rule" is outdated and should be modified or eliminated for qualified primary care networks and integrated health care delivery systems that demonstrate financial soundness and management ability. Similarly, the Medicaid freedom of choice provisions for managed care plans are outdated and inconsistent with options available to other participants in primary care networks. Medicaid beneficiaries should have flexible provider selection within a network, and the freedom to opt out. However, for services available in the network, a Medicaid beneficiary must bear some costs for opting out.

Consideration must be given to the adequacy of reimbursement to rural, integrated health care delivery systems. Specifically, Medicare pre-paid managed care reimbursement is based upon the Adjusted Average Per Capita Cost methodology (AAPCC). AAPCC is inherently flawed as applied to rural networks. A more reasonable methodology needs to be developed. Similarly state Medicaid reimbursement rates need to be based on actual costs of providing services in rural areas. State and federal programs that transfer an inappropriate level of risk to rural, primary care networks threaten the viability of the fragile rural health care delivery system. Federal standards for reasonable and actuarially sound rate-setting should be considered, including adjustments for demographic characteristics and risk-selection by beneficiaries.

Successful community-based, primary care networks utilize managed care information techniques. Medicare and Medicaid information reporting should be standardized and made consistent with state-of-the-art managed care techniques developed in the private sector.

Other modifications to Medicare and Medicaid may also be desirable in order to expand participation in private-sector, rural primary care networks and integrated health care delivery systems. The rural health care system will be strengthened by such participation. However, such participation must be on terms that are consistent with the rigorous requirements that such systems meet in serving private sector employers and individuals.

*   *   *   *   *   *   *

I would like to close my remarks by noting that rural health needs can be met by private-sector, integrated health care delivery systems and their community-based, primary care networks. Rural areas are as different from each other as they are generally different from urban areas. If health care legislation leaves enough flexibility for local solutions to be devised, rural residents will be able to receive high quality health care at reasonable cost.

We would be happy to work with the Committee and its staff in designing reform legislation that encourages local solutions to integrated health care delivery systems in rural areas.

PREPARED STATEMENT OF HEIDI HARTMANN

I am Heidi Hartmann, Director of the Institute for Women's Policy Research; I am a labor economist and hold the Ph.D. degree from Yale University. I want to thank you, Chairman Moynihan, Senator Bradley, and other members of the Committee on Finance for the opportunity to testify before you today. It is a pleasure to share our new research findings with you at this important hearing on underserved populations and health care reform.

My testimony today is based on our forthcoming report on women's access to health insurance, which presents findings from the first thorough study of the factors that affect women's access and lack of access to health insurance. It shows that certain groups of women fall through the cracks of our current health care system. These women do not have access to health insurance either through their employers, spouses, or the public system, nor can they purchase insurance themselves. Without health insurance, these women are chronically underserved. Our forthcoming report also assesses how well President Clinton's proposed Health Security Act would address women's inadequate access to health insurance.

Among the groups of women particularly at risk of having no insurance are women of child bearing age, single women and single mothers, women with low educational attainment and low income, women of color, and women undergoing transitions in marital or employment status. In addition, women who work part-time, in low wage jobs, in small firms, and/or in certain industries that employ women disproportionately are especially likely not to have health insurance provided by their employers and to be uninsured as a result.

Our study, conducted by a team of five IWPR researchers, relies on data collected by the Census Bureau in its monthly Current Population Survey of 60,000 households which are representative of the nation's population. Our team used the public use tapes from January and March of 1991, the most recent time period for which data on job tenure are available. The study was supported by the Henry F. Kaiser Family Foundation as part of the Kaiser Health Reform Project.

We focus on women's access to health insurance for several reasons. Women are a large proportion of the population, the majority in fact, yet their specific needs are often overlooked in public policy debates. Women also have a unique relationship to the health care system. Recent studies show that women use health care services more than men do and spend a greater portion of their income on health care. In addition to having significant personal health needs, women facilitate use of the health care system by other family members, and, in particular, are responsible for the family planning and pre- and post-natal care crucial to the birth and rearing of healthy children.

The way women obtain health insurance differs from men as well. Because women's relations to family and work tend to differ from men's (basically women do more family care and men do more paid work), women are more likely to have *indirect* access to employment-based health insurance (access as a dependent covered by a worker's policy) and less likely to have *direct* access through their own employment. In other words, traditionally women have relied on their husbands' jobs to provide them with health insurance. We believe this traditional reliance places women at increased risk of being uninsured over significant and growing portions of their lives.

Already the majority of women do not receive their health insurance indirectly through husbands and this majority will only grow larger in the future. As women continue to marry later and divorce more, increasing numbers of women will be unmarried for longer portions of their lives and will not have access to health coverage through husbands. In addition, as the proportion of child birth occurring outside marriages continues to increase, women increasingly need direct access to health insurance. Even within marriages, women can no longer be sure that their husbands will receive insurance through their employers, especially insurance that provides coverage to other family members at reasonable cost, as jobs decline in industries such as manufacturing that have traditionally provided generous benefits and increase in sectors that provide fewer full-time regular jobs with only limited fringe benefits at best. The proportion of adults obtaining insurance through employment, both directly and indirectly, has been falling since at least 1988. Given the changes underway in family structure and employment, women have an increased need for secure access to insurance.

For these reasons, we believe it is especially important to examine women's access to direct employer-provided coverage and to understand the difficulties women face in obtaining insurance through their own employment. Figure 1 shows that women are much less likely to have direct employer-provided insurance than men, 37 percent versus 55 percent. Women's greater access to indirect coverage (28 percent for women versus 10 percent for men) makes up the difference, while women's greater access to public insurance means that overall a somewhat smaller proportion of women are uninsured than men (15 percent of adult women versus 19 percent of men). Women are fortunate in having access to more sources of insurance than men, but their greater reliance on indirect coverage through their spouses leaves many women vulnerable to life cycle events such as leaving the parental home, divorce, widowhood, or the retirement or job loss of a spouse.

Overall, we identified three types of issues that affect women's access to health insurance: life cycle factOrs factors related to social and economic status, and factors related to the extent and type of employment women have.

LIFE CYCLE FACTORS

Women need more health care during young adulthood, the peak child bearing years, yet, as can be seen in Table 1, women under 30 are substantially more likely to be uninsured. Young adults, 18-20, obtain most of their health insurance indirectly through their parents, which they then lose as they leave home and school. Women in their twenties are especially unlikely to have access to indirect insurance through parents or a spouse's job. The lack of insurance in this age range is especially troublesome, as 70 percent of all births in 1990 were to women under age 30. Young adults, under age 25, whether male or female, often do not have strong job attachment and so are less likely to have employer-provided insurance. They experience more job change as well as more unemployment. Our study shows that uninsurance falls for both women and men as they age and that, at all ages, men have more direct insurance than women. Men also are more likely than women to lack insurance at all ages (because, in comparison with women, they have less access to insurance through spouses' jobs and less access to public insurance).

Table 1 also shows that married women with spouses present have the most insurance, because of their high access to indirect insurance (still, less than a majority, 43 percent, of married women receive their insurance through their spouses). Women in all other marital status categories (married with absent spouse, separated, divorced, widowed, or never married) are twice as likely to be uninsured. And women most likely to be experiencing marital transition (those in the spouse absent and separated categories) have the highest rates of uninsurance (24 percent, not shown on table). We also found that married women whose spouses work less than full-time, full-year are just as likely to have no insurance (18 percent) as those whose spouses do not work at all, whereas only 8 percent of those with spouses employed full-time, full-year lack insurance (not shown on table).

Among women with children, those who are single parents are especially likely to be uninsured (18 percent lack insurance compared to 11 percent of mothers in two-parent families), even though Medicaid targets poor single mother families. The highest rate of direct employer-provided insurance is found among women who have no children (41 percent).

The great disparities in insurance rates between married women whose husbands work full-time year-round, other married women, unmarried women, young women, and single mothers indicate that our system is based on assumptions that do not work for all women. We must question the adequacy of a social system that leaves women who need health care most, specifically those in the child-bearing years, the least likely to have health insurance.

RACE, EDUCATION, AND FAMILY INCOME

Social and economic factors also greatly affect which women have access to health insurance. As shown in Table 1, women of color are approximately twice as likely as non-Hispanic white women to lack insurance, with Hispanic women being nearly three times as likely as white women to be uninsured. African American women have especially low access to health insurance through husbands (only 10 percent compared to 31 percent for white women).

Women with low levels of education and low family income are also disadvantaged by our current system. Women with less than a high school diploma are twice as likely to be uninsured as high school graduates and women with low family income (less than $15,000) are more than five times more likely than women in moderate and higher income families to be uninsured (32 percent versus 6 percent). It is clear that public insurance does not close the insurance gap for women in low-income families. In the $15,000–$25,000 income range, the range in which the median single mother family falls, about one in five women lack insurance (not shown on table). Like insurance coverage generally, women's direct coverage (through their own employer) increases with educational attainment and family income. Nearly three times as many college graduates as high school dropouts have direct employer-provided health insurance.

It is clear that the current employer-based system fails to serve women in low-income families and women of color.

THE EXTENT AND TYPE OF WOMEN'S EMPLOYMENT

Women's access to insurance through employment is greatly affected by the nature of the jobs they hold—their hours of work, years on the job (tenure), earnings, and the firm size and industry of their employers, among other factors. Among women workers, women have less access to direct employer-provided health insurance at least partly because they are disproportionately located in industries or types of employment in which employers traditionally do not provide insurance. Women also have' less direct employer provided health insurance even when they work in the same types of jobs as men do.

Table 2 shows that for virtually all the work-related characteristics studied, men have more direct insurance than women while women have more indirect insurance and less uninsurance than men. Direct employer provided insurance is rare among women working part-time, fewer than 35 hours per week, but women with these low work hours are fortunate to have substantial indirect access through their spouses' jobs. While men working low hours have more direct access, they have very little indirect access through their wives' jobs and are thus more likely than women overall to be uninsured. Workers in the first year on the job, both female and male, have less direct insurance than those with longer job tenure, as do those who report having had some unemployment. While it is not surprising that workers who show less work attachment have less direct employer-provided insurance, it is surprising that women workers have even less coverage than similarly situated male workers. For women, then, transitions in employment present special difficulty in getting direct insurance.

Characteristics of the employer also affect the likelihood of having direct insurance coverage. In small firms and in the six industries that provide the lowest rates of coverage, men have more direct coverage than women have (except in construction). Differences between men and women in direct coverage are especially large in personal services and retail trade, and in the business/repair and entertainment services. Even women's greater indirect access still often leaves them with very high rates of uninsurance—particularly in small firms, and in personal services, retail trade, and agriculture. Those working in agriculture have the lowest rates of insurance through a spouse, likely reflecting the lack of alternative types of employment in rural areas that could provide access to health insurance.

Figure 2 illustrates differences in direct coverage for women and men by weekly work hours, years on the job, and firm size. Only 1 in 8 women working less than 25 hours per week has employer-provided health insurance, 2 in 5 women in the first year on the job have direct coverage, and only 1 in 4 of those working in small firms does.

In our study we also used multivariate statistical techniques to consider the effects of all these variables simultaneously, checking for effects that might be masked by other variables and determining which factors remain important. This analysis generally confirmed the importance of the variables discussed, showing most to be statistically significant determinants of health insurance coverage for women (and men).

IMPACT OF THE HEALTH SECURITY ACT

Our study points to many gaps in coverage in the current health care system. Therefore, we also considered the impact of health care reform on coverage for both women and men, modelling the effect of the President's Health Security Act, especially the proposed employer mandate. An employer mandate, particularly one covering all employers and all their employees, overcomes a number of barriers to insurance coverage. Women workers would overcome barriers to health insurance including low wages, short job tenure, low hours of work, and firms with low coverage rates.

Using data from the March 1991 Current Population Survey pertaining to 1990, we estimate how many employees, both male and female, not covered by their own employer would become directly insured under the Clinton plan (which requires employers to provide coverage for all those working at least 10 hours per week). Next we examine the resulting changes in the source of insurance coverage for men and women affected by the Clinton plan, estimating the numbers of workers who would be newly eligible to receive direct coverage who currently use indirect coverage or other private or public insurance, or are uninsured. We also explore how the new access to direct coverage varies by firm size, industry, and earnings levels. This analysis allows us to address how the burden of coverage would likely shift among employers and the impact that exempting small firms would have on the number of employees who would receive coverage.

We estimate that 29 million more women, or 50 percent of all working women, would have access to direct coverage from their own employer than now do so. Some 27 million men, or 40 percent of all working men, would be newly eligible for direct employer-based health care coverage. This access would reduce the risk of insurance loss from life cycle transitions in living arrangements that women (and men) currently experience. Nonworking adults married to those working for employers who are not currently providing insurance would also be newly covered indirectly through their spouses employment (we were not able to estimate this number). Among newly eligible male workers, 44 percent (11.9 million) would gain new coverage because they are currently uninsured, while 25 percent would switch from indirect coverage through a spouse (or parent). Among newly eligible female workers, only 27 percent (8 million) would gain new coverage while 46 percent would switch from indirect coverage.

Some working women and men, approximately 1.2 million women and fewer than 400,000 men, would still not have access to employment-based coverage, when the 10 hour screen is applied. In addition, many Americans, primarily those not working, will still need to obtain insurance through other payment means. Our data indicate that of the 26 million men and women currently without insurance, 20 million would gain direct coverage leaving 6 million working age men and women (ages 18-64) ineligible to receive direct employer-based coverage (see Figure 3). As noted above, some of these individuals may be eligible for indirect coverage as a currently uninsured spouse or parent gains access to direct coverage through the employer mandate. And, under the Clinton plan, which guarantees universal access, others, such as the unemployed, would purchase insurance as individuals, receiving subsidies according to their family income level, or would participate in an expanded public program.

Because the President's plan requires nearly all firms (all those with fewer than 5000 employees, employing about 85 percent of all workers) to participate in health insurance purchasing cooperatives, or alliances, women and men would be subject to much less change in their sources of health care when they experience transitions such as job change, job loss, leaving their parents' home, marriage, divorce, separation, or widowhood than they typically are now. Whatever the source of the payment for their health insurance (whether by their employer, themselves, or via subsidies or public programs), they would have the option of maintaining access to the same health care plan (of course, if they have to take on a greater share of the cost because of lack of employment they might choose to switch to a less expensive plan). In addition, women and men would have secure access for their dependents, since all employers, including those large firms not required to participate in the alliances, would be responsible for contributing their share (80 percent under the President's proposal) of the cost of coverage for dependents.

When we consider which employers would newly be required to contribute for their employees, we observe some surprises. Of the 29 million women who would be newly eligible to receive insurance through their own employers, the largest share, 13 million or 46 percent, are currently working for firms with 100 or more employees, 12 million or 41 percent are working for firms with fewer than 25 employees, and only 3.8 million or 13 percent work for firms employing 25 to 99 employees (see Figure 3). About half of the women newly eligible for direct coverage are employed either in retail trade (8.1 million) or professional service industries (7.9 million). In these industries, about half of the gains would be for workers in large firms, those with 100 or more employees. In contrast, in personal services most of the new access to direct employer-based insurance among women workers would occur in small firms, those with fewer than 25 employees.

For men compared to women, more of their new access is concentrated in the smaller firms. This is especially true for the construction industry. Among those construction workers who would become newly eligible for direct coverage, about 75 percent work in small firms. Of all 27 million male workers who would newly gain direct access, 14 million, Are than half, are currently working for firms with fewer than 25 employees, 9.4 million or 35 percent are working for firms with 100 or more employees, and 3.6 million or 13 percent work for firms with 25 to 99 employees.

A profile of the currently uninsured workers who would gain direct access to health insurance for the first time under a Clinton-style mandate shows that out of 7.7 million currently uninsured women workers, 5.8 million women (75 percent) earn less than $12,000, another 1.4 million (18 percent) earn between $12,000 and $23,999, and only 500,000 women (6 percent) earn over $24,000 (see Figure 3).

Our analysis shows that more of the working men (than women) who would be newly eligible for direct coverage come from the ranks of the uninsured, partly because they are less likely to be able to rely on their spouses' employers or public insurance. Out of these 12 million currently uninsured working men, 6.7 million (55 percent) earn less than $12,000, another 3.6 million (30 percent) earn between $12,000 and $23,999, id only 1.6 million (14 percent) earn over $24,000 (see Figure 3).

Thus, when women and men are considered together, nearly 80 percent of those who would become newly insured under a Clinton-style employer mandate earn less than $24,000 per year, and nearly 2/3 earn less than $12,000 per year. An employer mandate would bring health insurance coverage to substantial numbers of low-earning uninsured workers. In addition, nonworking dependents in their families would also become eligible for coverage through a mandate that requires coverage for dependents as well as workers (as the Clinton plan does).

Finally, we considered the effect on coverage for the uninsured if smaller firms are exempted from an employer mandate. Using the 10 hour screen from the Clinton plan, our estimates show that, out of all 26 million uninsured adults, 20 million uninsured workers would gain new direct insurance coverage under a universal mandate, compared to only 10 million if firms with fewer than 25 workers were exempted, and only 7 million would if firms with fewer than 100 employees were exempted (see Figure 3). These data indicate that plans which exempt certain firms from the employer mandate fail to cover many workers as well as nonworkers. If universal access is guaranteed, as it is in the Health Security Act, then the burden of covering workers in exempted firms will fall elsewhere in the system, for instance on the federal government.

In conclusion, our study shows that many women have inadequate access to health insurance in our current system. The assumption that all nonworking women or women with marginal employment can gain access to insurance through their husbands or parents is not supported by the facts.

Women have less direct access to health insurance through employment than men, 37 percent versus 55 percent or 29 million versus 42 million, and for many groups of women, neither indirect access through men nor public insurance makes up the difference. Many young women, women in transition out of marriages, and women whose husbands have employment that does not provide health insurance are at greater risk of being without insurance of any kind. I-ow income women, women with low educational attainment, and African-American and Hispanic women also lack insurance in disproportionate numbers. Our current employment-based system provides less insurance to low earners, part-time workers, and those on the job less than a year; many small firms and both large and small firms in particular industries also do not now provide health insurance to their workers. These differences not only raise questions about fairness, but also point to the undesirable society-wide outcomes that result from our current system of voluntary employer contributions to health insurance costs. Is it acceptable that women are least likely to have health insurance during their child bearing years, for example?

Our study shows that reform that includes an employer mandate would address many of the problems in health insurance access that women currently face. The failure of many employers to provide insurance disproportionately affects women.

Women have a greater stake in the outcome of the debate over employer responsibility, since they currently have less access to direct-employer provided coverage. An employer mandate like that proposed in the Clinton Administration's Health Security Act would bring direct coverage to 21 million women and 15 million men who now have other sources of insurance as well as new direct coverage to 20 million working adults, or three-fourths of all adults who are now totally uninsured. Among adult women aged 18 to 64, an employer mandate for those working more than 10 hours per week would provide new direct coverage to 8 million, or two-thirds of all uninsured women, according to our estimates. Among adult men, 12 million, or more than four-fifths of all uninsured men, would be newly eligible for direct employer-provided health insurance according to our estimates. In addition, some portion of the uninsured who are not working but are dependents of newly covered workers would also be eligible for health insurance as family members.

If the smaller firms are exempted from an employer mandate, the proportion of the uninsured who would gain new direct coverage would fall dramatically. When all firms are included, three-fourths of the uninsured gain direct coverage; if firms with fewer than 25 workers are excluded, the proportion falls to about two-fifths; and if those with fewer than 100 workers are excluded, the proportion getting new coverage falls to about one quarter.

As discussed above, an employer mandate would provide new direct coverage to many workers who are currently uninsured or who have access only indirectly through a spouse or a parent. Having direct access can protect many women from losing insurance as the result of reaching adulthood, family break-up due to divorce or separation, or the job loss of the insured. Having greater access to insurance from their own employers can thus provide greater security to women undergoing transitions in their family arrangements. Under the Health Security Act, which goes beyond an employer mandate by also guaranteeing universal access, workers also do not have to fear loss of insurance when they change jobs, experience unemployment, or leave the labor market for a period of time.

Despite almost complete reliance on employer provided coverage, the United States is alone among industrial countries in allowing employers absolute latitude as to whether, how, and to whom to provide health insurance coverage. As our research shows, a system where choice is left to individual employers leaves many people underserved.

Table 1: How Do Women Get Their Health Insurance?

(Women Ages 21-64) a

Characteristics	Total		Percent Distribution			
	Number (in thousands)	Percent b	Direct %	Indirect %	Other %	Uninsured %
BY AGE						
18-20	5,303	100	10	42	26	22
21-24	7,324	100	31	16	30	23
25-29	10,436	101	43	20	20	18
30-64	55,225	100	39	30	18	13
BY MARITAL STATUS						
Married, Spouse Present	45,622	100	33	43	14	10
All Other	27,363	99	48	1	29	21
BY PRESENCE OF CHILDREN & FAMILY TYPE c						
Single Parents	8,622	100	36	1	45	18
In Two Parent Families	24,608	101	30	47	13	11
Not Parents (Single and Married)	45,058	99	41	23	19	16
BY RACE						
White, Non-Hispanic	54,754	100	40	31	17	12
Afro-American, Non-Hispanic	8,799	99	39	10	30	20
Hispanic	5,859	100	28	19	21	32
Other Races, Non-Hispanic	2,624	100	33	22	27	18
BY EDUCATION						
Less than High School	11,796	100	19	20	33	28
High School	30,414	99	37	30	18	14
Some College	15,799	100	42	28	19	11
College or More	14,975	100	54	26	13	7
BY FAMILY INCOME d						
Less than $15,000	14,900	100	18	4	46	32
Between $15,000 - $30,000	17,319	101	43	22	18	18
More than $30,000	40,766	100	45	38	11	6
ALL ADULT WOMEN (21-64)	72,985	101	39	27	20	15

Notes: a Except as otherwise noted.

    b Percents may not add to 100 due to rounding.

    c Ages 18-64.

    d Family income pertains to the 1990 calendar year.

Source: IWPR analysis of data from the 1991 March Current Population Survey.

Table 2a: How Do Employed Women Get Their Health Insurance?

(Employed Women Ages 21-64)

Characteristics	Total		Percent Distribution			
	Number (in thousands)	Percent a	Direct %	Indirect %	Other %	Uninsured %
BY HOURS PER WEEK b						
Less Than 24	7,754	99	13	47	23	16
Between 25-34	5,734	99	24	35	22	18
At least 35	40,491	101	62	16	11	12
BY JOB TENURE c						
Less than 1 year	3,234	100	41	24	16	19
Between 1 and 10 years	10,604	100	57	23	10	10
At least 11 years	3,879	100	70	17	7	6
BY UNEMPLOYMENT b						
Those who reported unemployment	7,776	100	35	22	20	23
Those who did not report unemployment	46,202	100	53	23	12	12
BY ANNUAL EARNINGS b						
Lower Wage Workers (< $15,000)	27,584	100	29	30	21	20
Higher Wage Workers (> $15,000)	25,907	100	74	14	7	5
BY FIRM SIZE d						
Less than 25 Employees	14,732	100	23	33	23	21
Between 25 and 99 Employees	6,560	101	48	23	14	16
At least 100 Employees	32,687	100	64	18	9	9
BY INDUSTRY d,e						
Agriculture/Forestry	705	100	21	23	33	23
Construction	741	100	47	26	11	16
Retail Trade	9,427	100	31	27	20	22
Business/Repair Services	3,035	100	35	29	18	18
Personal Services	3,206	100	19	27	25	29
Entertainment Services	545	100	31	30	23	16
ALL WOMEN WORKERS	53,978	101	51	23	14	13

Notes: a Percents may not add to 100 due to rounding.

  b Refers to 1990 calendar year.

  c Refers to jobs held in January 1991. A smaller data sample consisting of matched data from the January and March
  Current Population Surveys was used for this analysis.

  d Refers to longest job held in 1990.

  e Six industries with lowest rates of direct employer coverage.

Source: IWPR analysis of data from the 1991 March Current Population Survey.

Table 2b: How Do Employed Men Get Their Health Insurance?

(Employed Men Ages 21-64)

Characteristics	Total		Percent Distribution			
	Number (in thousands)	Percent a	Direct %	Indirect %	Other %	Uninsured %
BY HOURS PER WEEK b						
Less than 24	2,389	100	20	14	35	31
Between 25-34	2,504	101	25	11	26	39
At least 35	58,452	100	66	8	10	16
BY JOB TENURE c						
Less than 1 year	3,019	100	52	11	13	24
Between 1 and 10 years	11,429	100	68	9	8	15
At least 11 years	6,461	100	78	6	10	6
BY UNEMPLOYMENT b						
Those who reported unemployment	10,600	100	41	9	14	36
Those who did not report unemployment	52,745	100	67	8	11	14
BY ANNUAL EARNINGS b						
Lower Wage Workers (< $15,000)	17,409	100	30	10	20	40
Higher Wage Workers (> $15,000)	45,604	100	76	7	8	9
BY FIRM SIZE d						
Less than 25 Employees	19,587	100	35	13	21	31
Between 25 and 99 Employees	8,456	100	63	8	8	21
At least 100 Employees	35,301	100	78	5	8	9
BY INDUSTRY d, e						
Agriculture/Forestry	2,413	100	23	11	30	36
Construction	7,284	100	43	12	13	32
Retail Trade	8,252	100	49	9	16	26
Business/Repair Services	4,439	100	49	11	14	26
Personal Services	1,306	100	46	10	16	28
Entertainment Services	841	100	45	8	21	26
ALL MEN WORKERS	63,345	100	63	8	12	17

Notes: a Percents may not add to 100 due to rounding.

b Refers to 1990 calendar year.

c Refers to jobs held in January 1991. A smaller data sample consisting of matched data from the January and March Current Population Surveys was used for this analysis.

d Refers to longest job held in 1990.

e Six industries with lowest rates of direct employer coverage.

Source: IWPR analysis of data from the 1991 March Current Population Survey.

⇨ **Women have less access to health insurance from their own employers (direct-employer based) than do men.**

⇨ **Considering all sources, men have slightly less health insurance than women.**

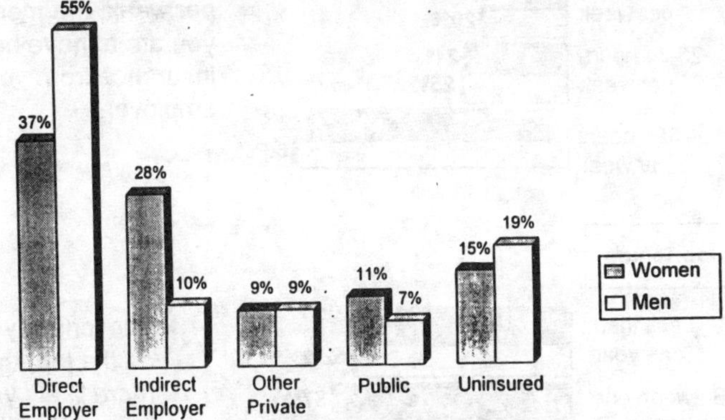

Source: IWPR analysis of data from the March 1991 Current Population Survey

Figure 2. Direct - Employer Based Coverage for Employees Ages 21-64 by Gender, Hours Worked Per Week, Firm Size, and Job Tenure

Percent with Health Insurance from Own Employer

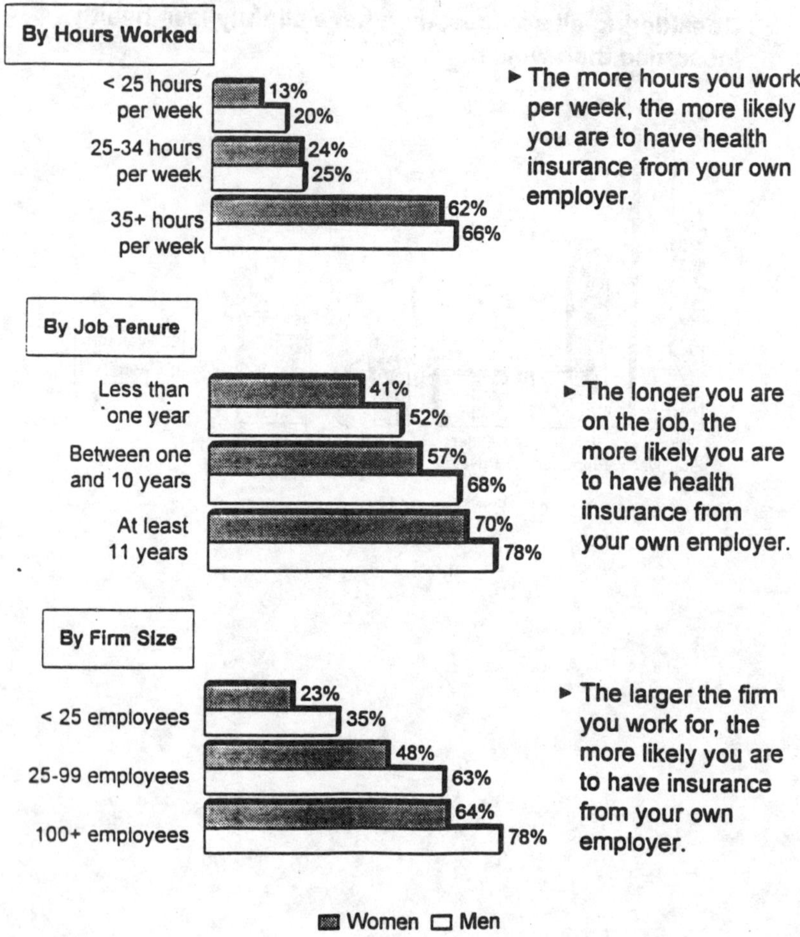

Source: IWPR analysis of data from the March 1991 Current Population Survey.

Figure 3. Impact of Health Security Act on Workers Aged 18-64

Number of Workers (in Millions) Gaining Health Insurance from Own Employer

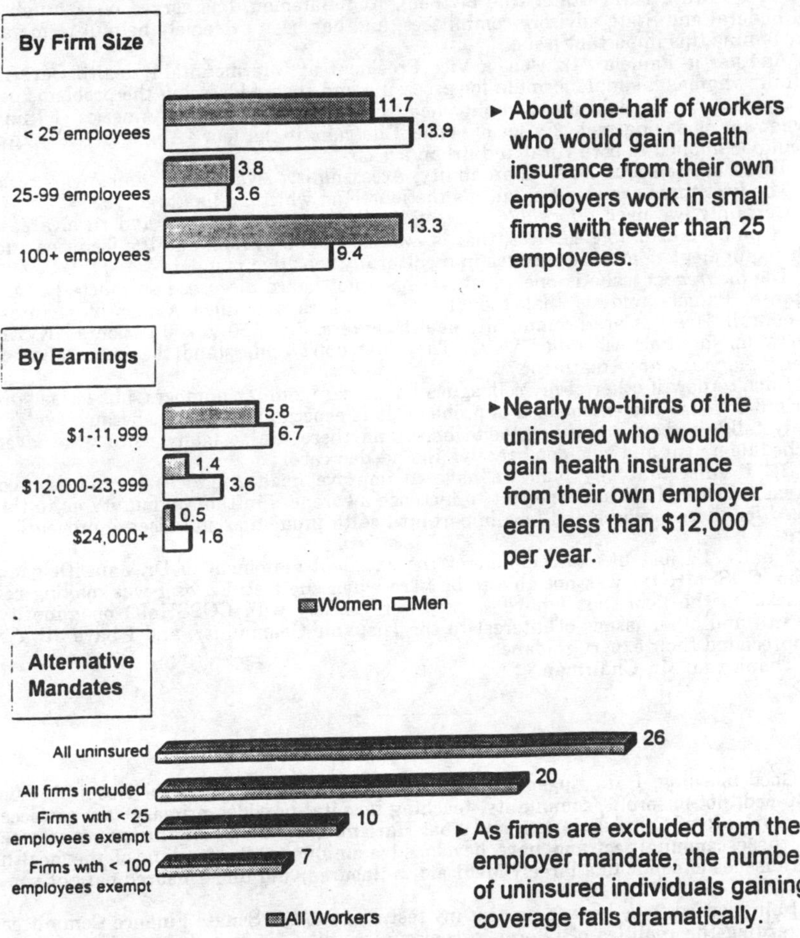

▶ About one-half of workers who would gain health insurance from their own employers work in small firms with fewer than 25 employees.

▶ Nearly two-thirds of the uninsured who would gain health insurance from their own employer earn less than $12,000 per year.

▶ As firms are excluded from the employer mandate, the number of uninsured individuals gaining coverage falls dramatically.

Source: IWPR analysis of data from the March 1991 Current Population Survey.

Prepared Statement of Senator Orrin G. Hatch

Mr. Chairman: I will keep my remarks brief, as I know we have a lot of witnesses this morning.

We have a number of rural health care experts in Utah, as you might imagine, since we are a rural State. One of them, Ken Bateman, has served on a number of Federal and State advisory committees, and has been extremely helpful to me as I examine this important issue.

Another is Pamela Atkinson, a Vice President at Intermountain Health Care in Utah, who has a simple formula for assessing and then addressing the problems associated with the delivery of quality health care services in rural America. I think what she is saying makes a lot of sense. She calls it the four "A"s, and really this could be applied to both rural and urban areas.

These are the four "A"s: Affordability; Accessibility; Availability, and Awareness. The first three are obvious, but it's the fourth on which I'd like to focus.

Certainly, we need *affordable, accessible* services in both urban and rural areas. And we need *available* services, that is, we need the providers and the facilities and the equipment to provide services in a culturally sensitive manner.

The *awareness* issue is one which we have not heard discussed as much. For instance, Pamela told us that they have 950 visits scheduled a month in Intermountain Health Care's community health centers. But, 150 to 200 patients NEVER show up for their scheduled visits. They just don't understand the importance of early diagnosis and treatment.

I don't know if other of my colleagues have heard similar numbers, but I was surprised to learn the extent of this problem. It is especially troubling, because we are only talking about *scheduled* visits here, and there are so many more who never schedule a visit and who don't receive the needed care.

So, I think that any plan we have to improve health services in underserved areas, must include a component to increase awareness in the community as to the need for these services and how important health promotion and disease prevention are.

Finally, I'd just like to compliment the excellent statement of Dr. Jane Delgado from COSSMHO; I was not able to be here when she testified as I was making remarks on the floor, but I have worked very closely with COSSHMO on minority health and other issues of interest to the Hispanic Community, and I have always appreciated their expert guidance.

Thank you, Mr. Chairman.

Prepared Statement of Eugene McCabe

Good morning. I am Eugene McCabe, President of North General Hospital. Our 240-bed, not-for-profit, community, teaching hospital provides primary care services to residents of Central Harlem and East Harlem. We have a long history of service in these communities, and have developed a unique understanding of the health care issues endemic to a largely Medicaid, uninsured, and underinsured patient population.

I am pleased to be here to present my testimony to the Senate Finance Committee regarding the realities of reform in communities like Harlem. I appreciate the opportunity to help identify those elements I believe must be considered in the design of standards for improved access to care—and to assist in defining the provisions for quality services that would be part of a reformed healthcare landscape.

As we view the progress of healthcare reform, it appears certain that the final bill will be constructed from a variety of elements shared by the administration, the House and the Senate. But, no matter what the origin, we believe universal access is key to any reform package. We also strongly believe that the Essential Community Provider provision in the administration's bill should be strengthened to reflect the role physicians and hospitals serving communities like Harlem have played historically—and continue to play, despite many obstacles.

Each day, the media reports the inexorable movement toward the creation of networks by healthcare providers through merger, acquisition and/or affiliation. The underlying reasons for this consolidation which by the way we agree with, are projected to reduce cost and improve services. If indeed this is to be the brave new world of health care, providers in the Harlems across the country share basic concerns—Will their current role be compromised? Will they have the opportunity to participate in these networks? Will their unique relationship with their patients change?

Last Thursday, in a meeting with Harlem physicians at North General Hospital, Hillary Rodham Clinton heard first hand the concerns of minority providers regarding reform. The consensus at that meeting was that it would be inexcusable if a consequence of seeking to improve healthcare in Harlem was to lock out providers that have rendered quality service to this population for so long. But these concerns are expressed throughout New York City as well.

It is a fact that our City shoulders a large share of the nation's healthcare ills. For example, of the 37 million uninsured Americans, 1.5 million are New Yorkers. While the City's Medicaid and uncompensated care expenditures continue to grow exponentially, there has been no measurable improvement in health status—and it could get worse.

We must be frank, some computer models suggest a significant hit to New York City Hospitals under current estimates. Specifically, it has been projected that some reform measures could result in a $30 million loss for North General Hospital. If extrapolated over the vista of New York City Hospitals, we are talking about billions of dollars being drained from our already unstable system.

However, we clearly support the need for reform because each day we witness the ravages of a system where many are denied prompt and effective care. Our overused emergency rooms and under-utilized primary care services drive up costs creating instability in an already overburdened system.

Despite these dire predictions, we welcome change and the time for reform is now. We view this as an opportunity for North General and community physicians to participate in shaping the future of health care delivery in our neighborhoods.

Every day we see patients who only seek care when a chronic problem has escalated to an acute level. When this happens, care is often less effective and always more expensive. Last year at North General, we provided over 25,000 emergency department visits—the majority of these visits were to patients in need of basic primary care services. Moreover, the 100,000 ambulatory care visits we provide at the hospital could be better served by managed care in less expensive settings.

In anticipation of change, we have designed programs to link patients with primary care providers. We educate our patients about preventive care and how to access the system. And while we have done a lot of work in this area, much more remains to be done. Our patients' priorities are often something other than prevention. Any new delivery system has to consider the episodic manner in which they access care and its impact on their health and healthcare expenditures. North General is playing a leading role in the development of a service delivery network, organized to increase access, ensure quality and promote cost efficiencies. The network will integrate the services of hospital and community based physicians, a home health agency, a long term care facility and ambulatory care centers. By forming this network, these providers will assume fiscal and clinical responsibility for the provision of high quality services to our patients. At North General, we are currently a step ahead of the game. We operate a sophisticated management information system which will drive the network, share data and facilitate access to patient information.

It would appear that our network meets all the qualifications of an Essential Community Provider based on our history of service and the federal designation of our service area as a health manpower shortage area. What concerns us, however, is the level of support that will be provided for Essential Community Providers.

Limited grant awards have been offered in various proposals which, based on our experience, will fall short of the expenses associated with network development. Projected costs for primary care site development, management information systems, planning, staff recruitment, training, and health promotion far outstep proposed subsidies in an area where strategic investment can significantly reduce costs.

Additionally, funding for enabling services, (i.e., outreach, social services, translators, transportation) required of grant supported Essential Community Providers, should not be provided through a separate mechanism. Instead, these services should be financed through the development grants. Furthermore, we believe that larger, better financed health plans that do not qualify for ECP funding must be required to provide enabling services if they choose to target these populations. This revision in the bill will level the playing field.

Hospitals and physicians that have served populations like ours have had limited access to capital for plant, equipment and management information system infrastructure. Grant funds and loans must be ample enough to support the development of these systems so that we can effectively compete with the large private health plans who will find our patients attractive once they have access to a health security card.

Reform has already caused shifts in the corporate structure of healthcare providers as they form delivery systems. It follows suit, then, that tax laws governing these providers should be amended to reflect this new healthcare environment and protect their 501(c)(3) status.

Current tax laws limit non-hospital providers to $150 million of tax-exempt debt. If not amended, this could effectively preclude many of the new systems from securing the additional tax-exempt financing required for network development. Forced to raise capital in the taxable market, providers will have to divert program funds for debt service.

Additional access points for primary care services will be required if we are serious about redirecting health utilization patterns. For providers in urban areas, tax incentives for capital formation are vital for expansion. This will be money well spent when you consider the savings associated with keeping people out of emergency rooms and inpatient settings.

It is clear that, at least initially, service to these populations will be more costly than that to the mainstream. Reform must recognize the fact that care to patients whose access has historically been compromised may require front end financing to put into place new and more efficient systems of care.

In closing, the health care market is already under reform. North General Hospital and other community health care facilities have dealt with issues of access, quality care and cost containment in low income communities long before reform became part of the public debate. We have weathered inadequate reimbursement methodologies, high costs from serving sicker patients that use the hospital for emergencies, and difficulty in retaining qualified physicians. We believe that improving these conditions is possible if reform recognizes that those who have been doing the job need new tools to compete in the new environment.

We wish to compete, we can compete, and we are confident that reform is the way to go. All we ask for are the tools to continue the task.

PREPARED STATEMENT OF CLYDE W. ODEN, JR.

I. INTRODUCTION

Good morning. I am Dr. Clyde W. Oden, Jr., President and Chief Executive Officer of the Watts Health Foundation, Inc. (WHF), and its health maintenance organization (HMO), United Health Plan. I have been employed by the WHF for almost 25 years, and have had the honor of being its President for the last 15 years. I have lived and raised my family in South Central Los Angeles for the last quarter of a century. I serve as Assistant Pastor of Emmanuel African Methodist Episcopal Church, which is also located in South Central Los Angeles.

My testimony this morning concerns health care services in the context of an urban/inner city environment, with special focus on the problems of access, quality, cost, special needs and health status. The context of these remarks is to also provide an additional perspective on the issues surrounding health care reform, and how public policy may be expressed in a manner that will most benefit the lives of the citizens of this country, with special considerations for those who live in rural and urban America.

My perspective may be unique in that I serve as the Chief Executive Officer of an "essential community provider," which is a Federally Qualified Health Center; a managed care plan through our Federally Qualified Health Maintenance Organization; and as a public policy advocate, having served as a volunteer consultant to Hillary Clinton's Health Reform Task Force.

II. WATTS HEALTH FOUNDATION, INC.

WHF is a non-profit health service organization founded in 1967 to provide innovative, low-cost, high quality health care to residents of Watts. WHF has a proven track record in effectively serving the poor, the uninsured, the underserved and special populations. WHF prides itself on its innovation, creativity and "going that extra mile" in providing services to a population that has been traditionally overlooked by mainstream health care systems. Today, WHF is uniquely composed of two operational systems that have garnered wide praise and have been models for organizations nationwide: Community Health Programs, which focus on operating WHF's federally qualified health centers; and United Health Plan, the organization's federally qualified Health Maintenance Organization.

Through its Community Health Programs, WHF has evolved to become one of the largest private providers of primary health care in Los Angeles County, annually serving over 125,000 clients with more than 250,000 encounters a year. WHF serves primarily individuals who have been increasingly disenfranchised by the mainstream health systems—"vulnerable populations" like the poor, the elderly, the immigrants, the addicted, the homeless, the chronically and terminally ill, and those without health insurance. With the support of a network of government and private grants, WHF serves these patients through an unique array of programs (over 30 programs) that have been woven together into a comprehensive service network. The population Community Health Programs serves is approximately 45 percent African American, 45 percent Latino, and the remaining 10 percent are Anglos and Asian Pacific Islanders.

The organization's HMO, United Health Plan, started in 1973 with an emphasis on the Medicaid population, but has evolved to include Medicare, employer-based markets, and a voluntary health alliance (Health Insurance Plan of California—HIPC). In California, United Health Plan is the tenth largest HMO and is the second largest HMO serving Medicaid beneficiaries. United Health Plan has nearly 100,000 members in Los Angeles, Orange, and San Bernardino counties. The dominate market remains those most vulnerable to issues of access and quality care, Medicaid recipients, which represents 69 percent of the membership. The Medicare market represents 16 percent, and the traditional (employer-based) commercial sector represents 14.5 percent of the membership.

History has shown us that out of despair, destruction and tragedy are born new beginnings, hope and progress. From the smoldering ashes of the 1965 Watts Riot rose the $6.5 million Watts Health Center—the new beginning that brought hope and progress to a devastated community. Following the riot in August 1965, the McCone Commission, a group appointed by then Governor Edmund G. Brown to investigate riot-torn areas in California during the 1960s. As a result of the McCone Commission's report, the South Central Multipurpose Health Services Center began in October 1967, as a federally funded demonstration project, with a $2.7 million grant from the Office of Economic Opportunity.

In 1970 the Center came under the administrative control of a community Advisory Council, who became it Board of Directors. In 1974 the Board renamed the organization the Watts Health Foundation, and in 1970 the Watts Health Center was completed. In 1973 the organization started its first prepaid health care program for Medicaid beneficiaries. In 1983 the United Health Plan became a federally qualified HMO, and in 1984 started one of the first HCFA risk contracts for Medicare beneficiaries.

III. THE URBAN CHALLENGE

Although, the nation, state and local governments are giving greater attention to serving the uninsured and poor, there is a serious void and lack of participation from ethnic communities. Organizations who serve populations that represent the largest proportion of the uninsured and poor, who are primarily based in urban cities, are not being sought as a viable resource. The health reform debate, in many instances, is being lead by politicians, bureaucrats and private corporations who have had little, if any, direct experience in serving the uninsured. The challenge is to insure that urban-based organizations who have traditionally served the uninsured, underinsured and publicly supported individuals, become active participants in the health care reform debate. As the major for-profit health insurance agencies, hospitals, private providers, HMOs and corporations continue what is increasingly perceived as a self-serving debate on their rightful role in a reformed health care system, elected and appointed officials have a clear moral imperative to represent the collective needs, values and voices of their urban constituents.

IV. PROBLEM STATEMENT

From our organizational perspective, there is a serious health care crisis in urban/inner city America. This crisis is due in part to disproportionate numbers of uninsured and underinsured residents (including family members of uninsured workers); lack of access to primary health care providers; and accountable medical delivery systems; the growing cost of health care and medical technology; unhealthy lifestyles, and poor health seeking behavior on the part of residents who find themselves absorbed by their struggle for day to day survival, which in more cases than not take precedent over their own individual health care and family's health.

V. ISSUES

In making the best use of my time today, I would like to concentrate on five key issues: accessibility, accountable medical delivery systems, lifestyle consequences, cost of care, and linkages of health providers. In my final comments I will discuss issues related to current health care reform proposals.

A. Accessibility

Reality today, in many inner city communities, is that there are limited choices as to where residents receive health care services. Even the availability public health centers, federally qualified health centers, free and community clinics, and private practicing primary care physicians who still accepts Medicaid payments, are limited and scarce in urban communities. In too many instances the use of hospital emergency rooms is the only option left. The result is the unacceptably high rates of infant mortality, high rates of preventable morbidity, and the chronic growth of health care costs.

Watts Health Foundation's approach to the problem of access is to locate facilities in proximity to the neighborhoods in greatest need, hire full time physicians and other health professionals to provide services in an efficient context, i.e. group practice, utilize 15 passenger vans to transport patients for appointments, and to reduce financial barriers through the use of sliding scale fees for low income residents.

Our organization pioneered the innovative concept of using mobile medical centers for health care delivery services. Poor public transportation, gang territories, and transient residents who lack knowledge of existing community resources combine to create a situation whereby it is more feasible to go to the patient, rather than waiting for the traditional practice of patient presenting to doctor. By setting up our mobile medical centers in school yards, in the parking lots of social agencies, churches, and local parks we have been able to reach persons who have been nearly invisible to conventional health systems.

It has been extremely helpful to recruit physicians and other health professionals through the National Health Services Corps. The Corps has been our primary means of increasing the number of capable and committed health providers who serve in many urban areas.

B. Accountable Medical Delivery Systems

We must go far beyond merely devising systems of appropriate payment to providers to address the health care problems in our urban/inner cities. *Systems of health care delivery must be responsible for the health status of its members, and there must be accountability.* The inappropriate use of emergency rooms, the low levels of childhood and adult immunizations, the lack of screening for breast and prostate cancers, the troubling presence of preventable and treatable diseases such as tuberculosis, sexually transmitted diseases, and the rapid spread of HIV infections calls for accountability—even more so than merely payment for needed services.

Our 21 years of experience operating a managed care system, and our 27 years of being a fee-for-service provider have convinced me that in the urban/inner city context, managed care is the superior accountable medical delivery system.

The challenge is how to appropriate cost effective health care to individuals and to communities that are struggling with adverse economic, social, and political realities. We find, based on our experience in California, for many persons, seeking health care services at the earliest appropriate time does not occur—unless they are being aggressively pursued by systems of care that are monitoring their health status.

Our experience further confirm that timely prenatal care, follow-up of immunizations, early intervention of diseases, and health screening have best been done by systems of care that understand the failure to change such behavior leads to increased costs because of preventable hospitalizations and prolonged illnesses.

We find that there is minimum institutional consequence when additional encounters and services are appropriately provided when our fee-for-service patients presents. On the other hand, our relationship with our prepaid patients is different. There are serious consequences when inappropriate health seeking behavior continue to exist for health plan members. Emergency room admissions lead to costly visits and sometimes inappropriate hospital admissions. Missed appointments for prenatal care leads to potentially expensive preterm or low weight infants, and uncontrolled hypertension may lead to costly rehabilitation as a result of strokes and cardiac problems. As a result, significant intervention by our HMO occurs in the life of our members to address the consequences of delayed or missed treatments.

In the former instance where the fee-for-service relationship exist, reminders of follow-up visits are often viewed as merely creating additional fee opportunities, however, in the latter case, there is a contract between the system and the patient, and reminders are expected and accepted because of that contractual relationship. The accountability makes a difference.

C. Lifestyle Consequences

Health status in any community is impacted as much by style as it is by the health services received. There is ample evidence to demonstrate that the stressors of living, especially in urban/inner city areas, have led to inappropriate life style choices. Whether the issue is poor nutrition, lack of exercise, excessive alcohol consumption, use of tobacco products, violence, use of illicit drugs, or other high risk behaviors, lifestyle choices impact health status.

In the context of the debate on health reform, the experience of the Watts Health Foundation may be instructive. Health care agencies must advocate in the community and to the consumer appropriate lifestyle behavior. This is not only good public policy, but it has economic consequences to accountable health systems, such as our organization. We have in place programs of nutrition—including a major WIC program, prevention and treatment programs for alcohol, drug and tobacco addiction, and health education programs designed to address and control the spread of sexually transmitted diseases—including HIV infections.

Our concentrated efforts on community and patient health education have led to better health outcomes for the populations we serve.

D. Cost of Care

Central to health reform is the issue of cost, both paying for existing services as well as impacting inflationary pressures on health care. Our track record, we believe, has demonstrated that managed care services can be provided in a cost effective manner to residents in urban/inner city communities. The conventional wisdom, prior to our experience, had been that managed care cannot be done effectively in our service area communities, and that costs cannot be controlled. Conventional wisdom is proven wrong in both instances.

Effective regulation of managed care, such as we now find in California through the Department of Corporations—the state regulatory agency for all HMOs, and the State Department of Health Services—which regulates Medicaid prepaid contracts, assures that appropriate corporate behavior is maintained. Although Medicaid is still painfully under-funded, and the premiums are too low, our organization has been able to grow and reinvest in its future with very thin margins.

On the other hand, in the private markets where we compete with more than two dozen other HMOs, the pressure of competition is driving rate increases closer to the general Consumer Price Index (CPU, and in some recent instances—under the CPI. This demonstration of market place competition is not only forcing costs down, but is forcing increased cost effectiveness within the managed care industry.

We find our organization looking to technology and creativity to keep our premiums competitive, because payors in the current California climate, have demonstrated quite convincingly that it is a buyer's market. Price regulations are not necessary, open market competition is a powerful incentive for lower cost.

E. Linkage of Health Providers

In this current debate on health reform, there has' been appropriate concern focused on how to include "essential community providers," "safety net providers," and "traditional providers": those physicians and other health care professionals who have been located in urban/inner city communities, and who have not generally been a partner in managed care systems. The question is how should these providers be included in health care reform.

It is our view that these providers, whether they be community health centers, minority providers, public health clinics and hospitals, should be given assistance to acquire levels of performance and expectations now to be required of managed care systems that are competing for patients in the greater metropolitan and suburban areas of our country.

In general these providers lack access to capital, staff and professional development, and technology development. Assistance in these areas is necessary to allow their inclusion as full partners in managed care systems, or in some instances, to enable them to compete with managed care systems. Concentrated efforts toward consumer education are necessary so that informed decisions can be made as greater health coverage is made available, and these systems of health care delivery becomes available.

Specifically, grandparenting of any class of providers into a managed care system, such as "any willing provider" clauses, or mandatory contracting for some classes of providers, will not—in my judgment—give these providers the standing necessary for long term survival in a reformed health system.

These providers have significant assets in loyal patients whom they have served well, and any managed care system seeking increased market share would gladly incorporate such providers into their systems. The problem is however, that many of these providers are not fully prepared to participate with managed care because their delivery service is oriented toward fee-for-service, and there has not been sufficient investment in infrastructure development to become fully integrated into managed care systems.

It is our recommendation that additional funding be directed at federally qualified health centers to both expand them and develop new ones to serve communities and populations that are still underserved. More importantly, however, new funds must be directed at infrastructure development, with particular focus on facility development, technology enhancements, Board of Directors development, staff development, and assistance in promoting capital accumulation so that risk can be assumed in serving the population they know, and have treated with such competence over the last 28 years.

Mandatory contracting will create an environment in which these organizations will not understand the urgency of becoming more competitive in a health reform era where competition on price, quality, and patient satisfaction will determine patient choice, and opportunities for contracting with managed care systems.

The same recommendation goes for publicly funded health centers, and community physicians. Resources must be made available so tat private practicing physicians can be encouraged to form group practices and to locate new facilities in medically underserved areas. These facilities need to reflect the present and future expectation of primary health care delivery in the context of group practice. Presently the banking and insurance industry provides no incentives for reinvesting in urban/inner city communities for physicians and other health providers who want to provide the very best for the residents of these communities.

Additionally, these providers must be prepared to contract with managed care companies, and oriented to prepaid health systems. Perhaps a plan that provides funding to medical schools, at institutions such as Howard University, Drew University of Medicine and Science, Meherry Medical College and Morehouse Medical School for the retraining of physician specialists to become primary care specialists, would be appropriate public policy.

VI. COMMENTS ON CURRENT HEALTH REFORM PROPOSALS

What is most important are the principles upon which the Administration's proposal is built. These principles will serve urban/inner city residents very well, if they are incorporated into whatever legislation this Committee recommends to the Senate. Central is universal coverage. Whether through employer mandate, or individual mandate, health care coverage must be a right for every American citizen—and every legal resident of our country. Implicit in this universal coverage is affordability and accessibility.

Secondly, health reform without assurance that preventive and primary health care is available within the communities in which our citizens live, is not true reform. Some type of "catastrophic coverage" would place the emphasis on health care repair, rather than prevention and early intervention. The later is not only most cost effective, but the best of public policy.

Thirdly, insurance reform is a must. No one should be denied health care coverage because of pre-existing conditions, and appropriate coverage must follow our citizens.

Fourth, emphasis on quality is paramount, and public accountability for quality is a necessity. In this regard, there is a need to index health care outcome reporting to the health status of persons entering into health systems. A major indicator of quality service is the demonstrated improvement in health status within an organization's patient population.

Fifth, managed competition, especially in the context of urban/inner city communities, is a reasonable expectation. And, open competition between health systems and providers for the loyalty and support of the citizenry, will promote the type of accountable medical delivery systems required. This type of competition will keep premiums low, quality and patient satisfaction high.

Finally, choice must be an integral part of any reform. When citizens are in a market place where informed choice of health systems and health providers can be made, patient satisfaction can be optimized. Additionally, choice provides encouragement for systems to be culturally competent, linguistically compatible, and member friendly. Having choices also increases the opportunity for community providers to be included, particularly when they have been prepared for the era of health care reform.

VII. CLOSING

In closing, I would like to thank the Senate Finance Committee for inviting me here to speak. I also wish to commend Chairman Moynihan for his support of Medicaid managed care. The interest and cooperative work of this committee on health care reform is gratifying and is contributing greatly to the overall health care reform debate.

___

PREPARED STATEMENT OF SENATOR DAVID PRYOR

Mr. Chairman, I am pleased to be a part of today's hearing on the subject of access to health care in urban and rural communities. The reform which is so desperately required of our health care delivery system will rely, in part, upon reforms in our methods for providing care to our nation's underserved areas. I

join my colleagues in welcoming our distinguished panel of witnesses this morning. I look forward to their insights into the strengths and weaknesses of the current health care delivery system. While my remarks will focus on the rural aspects of the access problem, I am interested, as well, in the access problems experienced in urban areas.

Mr. Chairman, this nation creates some of the finest doctors in the world.

The very brightest, the very best of our young people have historically been drawn to the practice of medicine. The medicine they practice is widely regarded as state of the art, high tech and definitive. Where access to the care of these fine doctors is guaranteed, in parts of urban and most of suburban America, their care is considered the very best to be had. It's shiny, it's impressive, it's loaded with the latest bells and whistles. It's the Cadillac of health care.

Now, you don't see many shiny Cadillacs on dusty, back-state roads. And, unfortunately, you don't see many of our fine doctors there either. We are spending somewhere beyond five billion dollars a year to train medical doctors, dollars that flow from the paychecks of rural as well as urban neighbors through contributions to Medicare . . . with additional billions of tax dollars collected from rural as well as urban areas going to support other aspects of the health care delivery system . . . and yet we continue to struggle with access problems in rural areas. Improving access to care in rural areas will require improving access to health care providers. At this time, we just don't have enough of them.

While almost 25 percent of this nation's population lives in non-metropolitan areas . . . and in Arkansas this figure is closer to 47 percent . . . only about 13 percent of patient-care physicians, and 7 percent of hospital-based physicians practice there. We see no more than about 6 percent of our recent residency graduates choosing rural practice. And the numbers are not much better for other health professionals. In 1985, 30 percent of physician's assistants were practicing in rural areas. By 1990, this percentage had fallen to 13 percent. Only 15 percent of registered nurses practice in rural areas.

While rural residents pay to educate our physicians and to support our health care system, wonder, frankly, whether rural areas receive an adequate return on this investment as the system is currently structured.

I look forward to our panelists' responses to these concerns.

___

PREPARED STATEMENT OF BERNARD SIMMONS

Chairman Moynihan and Members of the Senate Finance Committee. My name is Bernard Simmons, Member of the Board of Trustees of the National Rural Health Association and Executive Director of the Southwest Health Agency for Rural People, Tylertown, Mississippi. I am representing the National Rural Health Association whose membership is comprised of small, rural hospitals, community and migrant health centers, rural health clinics, primary care physicians, non-physician providers, educators and other rural health advocates.

The National Rural Health Association appreciates the opportunity to testify on the implications of national health reform on rural communities.

The National Rural Health Association urges serious consideration and passage of a health reform plan that ensures universal access to health care for all populations. NRHA distinguishes universal access from universal coverage by defining universal access as access to basic comprehensive primary health care services. In our estimation, providing a health care card and offering health care benefits does not go far enough to providing quality health care services. American citizens, particularly those in isolated rural and frontier communities, must have access to primary health care providers.

SOUTHWEST HEALTH AGENCY FOR RURAL PEOPLE'S SERVICE AREA

The Southwest Health Agency for Rural People, Inc. (SHARP) is a private, nonprofit corporation and a rural community health center located in Southwestern

Mississippi, 85 miles north of New Orleans, 94 miles south of Jackson, Mississippi and 85 miles from the Gulf Coast of Mississippi. Tylertown is a rural community of almost 59,000 citizens. SHARP serves all or parts of a five county area designated as health professional shortage areas, Walthall County, MS, Lawrence County, MS, Pike County, MS, Northern Washington Parish, Louisiana and Northern Tangipahoa Parish, Louisiana.

Last year, SHARP served 3,846 people, with 18,200 patient encounters. We have estimated an unmet demand of 32,000, with just over 12,000 persons who are going unserved. In Walthall County the unemployment rate is 7.8 percent, the per capita income is $7,263, the rate of poverty is 35.9 percent, and the infant mortality rate is 8.6 percent for the White population and 12.3 percent for the non-White population.

HEALTH SYSTEMS FINANCING ISSUES

The National Rural Health Association believes that there are two major issues in financing health systems reform that must be considered in implementing national health reform. These are: (1) how to finance the overall system and (2) how to pay for services as well as reimbursement focusing on the patient/provider relationship.

NRHA recommends that reform of the health system cannot take place by reducing Medicare. Rural areas, with their disproportionate number of elderly, will suffer inordinately with any decrease in Medicare funding.

The National Rural Health Association recommends continuing Medicaid disproportionate share hospital payments to those hospitals serving a disproportionate share of low-income patients during the five year transition period.

We also recommend not eliminating the Medicare adjustment for outpatient capital costs for rural and inner city health care facilities.

MEDICARE HISTORICAL BIASES

it is clear that historical biases in reimbursement to rural providers exist in our current health care system. Medicare pays rural providers up to 40 percent less than their urban counterparts for the same services. Costs for those services in rural communities are generally higher because rural providers cannot take advantage of economies of scale and many other reasons.

If a new national health system bases the federal budget and allocation of funds on historical experiences, rural providers and their patients will be put at further risk of losing critical health care resources and services. Tim Size, Executive Director of the Rural Wisconsin Hospital Cooperative illustrated the problems relating to the rural/urban Medicare differential, reform of the Medicare index, expanding Medicare rates to all payers and the consequences if all three situations occur simultaneously.

Using wage index data from the September 1, 1993 Federal Register, Size was able to demonstrate the competitive disadvantage of Sauk Prairie Memorial Hospital being on the wrong side of the Wisconsin River. By all accounts, the wage index was estimated lower by 20 percent, the adjusted labor was lower by 20 percent, the non-labor rate was 23 percent lower and the overall base payment was 21 percent lower.

In addition to the lower Medicare payment rates to rural hospitals, the Prospective Payment Assessment Commission has restated its position that the current system for determining the PPS wage index should be replaced by one which accounts for actual proximity to neighboring hospitals, as well as the institutions' occupational mix. However, it is our understanding that the Health Care Financing Administration is not in the position to adopt ProPAc's recommendation.

Another concern is a proposal that cost controls be applied by using Medicare rates to all payers.

For 1992–93, ProPAC estimates an aggregate Medicare margin of –9.9 percent. In 1991, Medicare (5.4%), Medicaid (1.6/00) and uncompensated care (4.8%) losses were equal to 11.8 percent of total costs for rural hospitals. Losses were covered with surplus payments from private insurers equal to 13.8 percent of total costs.

If the current gain from private payers becomes a loss comparable to that already born due to Medicare, the total hospital loss as a percentage of total is estimated at 11.8% + 5.4% or 17.2 percent. The only remaining source of revenue to offset this loss would be a couple of percentage points worth of non-operating revenue. As rural hospitals have already driven their costs down in order to compensate for current Medicare discriminatory payments, there is little to no flexibility left in their budgets.

The National Rural Health Association recommends that the wage index reflect the price of labor by reimbursing rural hospitals with a fair occupational mix adjustment.

The National Rural Health Association opposes the reduction in hospital marketbasket update for rural hospitals.

RURAL COMMUNITY-BASED HEALTH CARE SYSTEMS UNDER NATIONAL HEALTH REFORM

Federally Qualified Health Centers (FQHC), like the Southwest Health Agency for Rural People, are defined as essential community providers under the Clinton bill. It is critical that there be a mechanism that recognizes and maintains the contributions of essential community providers—those community-based providers who have established themselves and demonstrated their ability to provide access to health care services for residents of rural underserved areas. There must be assurances that essential community providers participate and be protected in payment agreements during the initial five year transition.

An amendment approved by the House Ways and Means Health Subcommittee protecting essential community providers did not provide for rural health clinics to receive cost-based reimbursement. The National Rural Health Association supports cost-based reimbursement for both federally qualified health centers and rural health clinics. It should be noted that the rural health clinics program is the forerunner and served as the model for the FQHC program. Rural health clinics were the first to be paid on a cost-based reimbursement basis in order to keep primary care clinics in rural and underserved areas financially viable. Rural health clinics, like FQHCs, provide millions of primary and preventive health care visits annually and must be sustained as an integral part of the rural health care delivery system.

The experiences of rural health clinics is another illustration of the inherent biases in historical payments to rural providers. Rural health clinic reimbursement has been artificially suppressed as a result of the placement of caps that were not increased for many years. Any future payments based on historical experience will continue to place rural providers in an untenable financial position.

REIMBURSING PRIMARY CARE PHYSICIANS UNDER NATIONAL HEALTH REFORM

Biases exist in the historical payment to rural primary care providers. The Medicare reimbursement for office visits are substantially lower than the cost of providing the services. Medicare fees simply do not begin to cover the time and material that it takes to serve rural elderly residents. NRHA is concerned about the Medicare fee schedule structure in that widely varying geographic schedules would continue the inherent biases in restrictive payment to primary care providers. Ultimately, access problems will arise for rural residents who live in alliances with low rates and/or high administrative costs.

The National Rural Health Association believes that higher payments for primary care services can be achieved through reconfiguring the conversion factor or through bonus payments rather than through changes in relative values. Moreover, alliances or states should be required to adopt a national resource based fee schedule, but allow the alliances or states to negotiate with providers regarding the conversion factor.

To further assist rural communities to recruit and retain primary care providers, physicians, nurse practitioners and physician assistants, the National Rural Health Association supports a Medicare bonus payment increase of 20 percent for primary care providers serving in a health professional shortage area. Moreover, Medicare bonus payments should continue for a period of ten years regardless of whether the areas continues to be designated as a health professional shortage area.

DESIGNATING ESSENTIAL COMMUNITY PROVIDERS

The National Rural Health Association supports the automatic designation of essential co-unity providers to include (1) hospitals that would qualify for a Medicare disproportionate share adjustment; (2) federally qualified health centers; (3) rural health clinics; (4) sole community hospitals; (5) hospitals that would qualify as a Medicare-dependent hospital; and (6) entities designated by the state governor through the state health plan.

These providers have established themselves and demonstrated their ability to provide access to health care services for residents of rural underserved areas. These providers have been providing the primary and preventive care services, along with necessary enabling services to ensure access to rural citizens. These essential community providers need to have stop loss and contracting protections—protecting them against financial risk.

CAPITAL INFRASTRUCTURE DEVELOPMENT

National health reform will require capital infrastructure development of community-based health care institutions. It will require expenditures for bricks and mortar, as well as systems transitions and acquisitions. It will require accessible and affordable funding, in debt and equity markets, for rural institutions, including community and migrant health centers, rural health clinics and small and rural hospitals.

Funds must be made available for loan and loan guarantees, interest subsidies and direct grants. Funding must be provided for planning and construction costs to convert existing facilities to other models where appropriate. Examples of these models include the Essential Access Community Hospital/Rural Primary Care Program and the Medical Assistance Facilities program.

Direct grants should be provided to community health groups and to qualified hospitals with urgent capital needs where emergency certification and licensure to entities are threatened with closure or loss of accreditation or certification of a facility or of essential services is a result of life of safety code violations or equipment failures.

The National Rural Health Association supports funding of loans and for rural health networks. However, in many isolated rural and frontier areas, networks may not be possible. Therefore, it is critical that funding for capital infrastructure projects also be provided to individual rural health care facilities.

HEALTH SYSTEMS WORKFORCE

Increases in incentives for primary care providing training for all disciplines is critical to rural areas. It is the hope of the rural constituency that greater emphasis on quality training at rural ambulatory, hospital and non-hospital sites will become a recruitment point for luring primary care physicians and non-physician providers to practice in rural communities.

NRHA supports direct graduate medical education reimbursement to rural ambulatory, hospital and non-hospital sites and paying of local providers for their time to teach.

The National Rural Health Association promotes a policy which adequately redirects graduate medical education payments to achieve a goal after a five year phase-in period of at least 50 percent of new physicians being trained in primary care rather than in specific specialty fields in which an excess supply currently exists.

Mr. Chairman, the National Rural Health Association is committed to working with the Congress and the President to ensure universal access through a national health reform plan this year.

PREPARED STATEMENT OF MARK SMITH

Good Morning. My name is Mark Smith, and I am Executive Vice President of the Henry J. Kaiser Family Foundation, an independent health care philanthropy with headquarters in Menlo Park, California. I am honored to be invited to speak with you today about the problems of "special populations" in health care reform.

I should state at the outset that I am here as an individual and that my statement does not necessarily represent the Foundation; furthermore, like the Foundation, I am not here to support or oppose any particular piece of legislation but, rather, to speak about this topic generally. You have several witnesses with you today who are more qualified than I to speak to the day-to-day problems facing low-income communities and their providers. Instead, I would like to address what I see as the main conceptual issues facing this committee as it considers the needs of special urban and rural populations.

I am a physician—a general internist, with much of my clinical and policy work for the last several years having been in the area of AIDS and HIV disease. I also hold an M.B.A. in Health Care Administration from the Wharton School at the University of Pennsylvania. Though like to think that this dual training and experience provides me with the compassionate, caring outlook of a physician and the practical, bottom-line orientation of a business person, I suppose it might be argued that my views represent rather than the best, the worst of both worlds: the self-serving, bleeding-heart sentimentality of health care providers and the flinty-eyed, steel-hearted, avariciousness of the health care merchant. So be it.

There are really two forms of "health care reform" going on in America today. Health Care Reform with a capital "R" is the sort being debated by both chambers of the Congress and by many state legislatures. This Reform concentrates on the financing of health insurance, and is considering broad expansion of coverage and methods to accomplish that expansion: employer and individual mandates, alliances, tax credits, underwriting reform, and the like. By health care reform with a small "r" I mean the changes going on in the real health care delivery system in the real world every day. This reform is far messier and less precise; but in some ways it is more profound than the debate which is capturing the headlines. Because of these changes, it is particularly important that Reform aimed at improving the circumstances of the underserved and vulnerable be aimed not at the problems of the old system as it was 10 or 15 years ago, but at those of the new system as it is today and will be tomorrow. In light of these changes, then, I would like to make 5 main points:

1. The health care system in America is changing dramatically and fundamentally.

The transformation sweeping across health care is being driven primarily by market forces, and is characterized by three features:

A. Increasing use of "managed care,"—"interventions in delivery and reimbursement of health care services . . . intended to reduce unnecessary or inappropriate care and reduce costs."[1]

B. Increasing aggregation of providers, both horizontally and vertically. Hospitals are merging. Medical groups are merging. HMOs are merging. Hospitals are buying medical practices. Insurance companies are buying medical groups. In its most advanced form, this trend is leading to "integrated systems of care" in which hospitals, physicians, home care agencies, and other providers are financially and organizationally linked.

C. Increasing use of capitation—pre-payment of a fixed amount of money—as the means by which providers are paid. This system, long a feature of staff and group model HMOs, is now extending to both primary providers and specialists in looser managed care arrangements as well.

To be sure, these developments are happening faster in some places than in others. But they are clearly the wave of the future throughout the country in the entire health insurance world. Indeed, a recent report by the Congressional Budget Office noted that one of the problems in studying cost savings from managed care compared to fee-for-service is that it is now virtually impossible to find traditional fee-for-service indemnity plans which have not adopted some of the features of managed care.

The trend toward managed care and capitation turns the traditional incentives of medical care upside down. In the old system, the more one did, the more one got paid. This approach has served the nation well in some ways but, it must be acknowledged, has also helped fuel the cost explosion in health. Indeed, we have the curious coexistence of undertreatment (for those who cannot pay) with substantial overtreatment (for those who can).

In the new system, providers are increasingly paid prospectively and the incentives are arrayed to perform more efficiently—that is to say, do less. This is a development which I welcome for many reasons. Not only does it provide forceful incentives to reduce costs by eliminating unnecessary treatment, but it also establishes for the first time the potential for a financial environment conducive to preventive care. Unfortunately, there is also a potential downside to this development: that the financial incentives on insurers and providers will lead to inadequate care or underservice.

Now, if you are relatively healthy and are socially and economically able to forcefully advocate for your interests should something untoward happen, this downside is probably outweighed by the fiscal and operational advantages of managed care. But there is, I believe, reason to be concerned if you are poor, non-white, or ill.

2. Getting to and affording health care is still a problem for many poor people.

Perhaps this should go without saying, but I will say it anyway. A study done for the Foundation by the National Opinion Research Center has demonstrated that, not withstanding the coverage provided by Medicaid, poor Americans continue to have substantial problems meeting their medical bills and paying medically-related expenses. Indeed, of the 10 problems ranked as most serious by Americans with household incomes less than $20,000, five are related to health, of which two are the financial responsibilities of paying for doctor or hospital bills (the highest ranking problem), or for prescription drugs (see Figure 1.)[2] And when NORC asked people about their ability to afford basic needs in the next year, concerns about medical bills outstripped concerns about clothing, food, and rent or mortgage. Indeed, low-income people cited these concerns about twice as often as Americans with incomes above $20,000 (see Figure 2).

3. The traditional providers for underserved populations are facing particularly perilous times.

Today's hearing focuses on "special populations" In what way might some Americans be "special" from the standpoint of the debate over health insurance reform? I can think of four moor ways: by virtue of having a low income; by virtue of geographic location (urban or rural) which has put them at a disadvantage; by virtue of being a person of color or of having difficulties with the English language or American culture, and, most ironically, by virtue of health status, that is to say they have difficulty with health insurance because they are sick.

Each of these groups represents a failure of the current market. All are served, to a greater or lesser extent, by system of public or quasi-public providers which has not been part of the changes in mainstream health care, and which is in increasingly desperate straits: public hospitals, voluntary hospitals in many big cities (such as New York) and rural areas, public health clinics, community and migrant health centers, a dwindling number of private doctors, and a very few managed care organizations. These providers rely heavily on Medicaid, state and local funding for the "medically indigent," and on categorically-funded programs such as those providing family planning services, prenatal care, and AIDS care: Title X, the Ryan White Care Act, the McKinney Act, and others. But one of the great ironies of the current situation is that these providers, most of whom have labored for years against great odds to serve the underserved and should be the most supportive of expanded insurance coverage, are among the most threatened by the changes happening in the market and contemplated by the Congress because, frankly, they would not be competitive.

The development of a new health care system (both the market-driven reforms and legislated financing and administrative arrangements) poses grave threats to the future of these institutions and programs. In this regard the transitional period from the old to the new will be a particularly tough one for them to negotiate, as they do not have many of the assets available to the private sector: management flexibility, capital reserves, access to capital markets. Furthermore, they will continue to struggle with the legacy of their past, which include's inferior physical plants, primitive information systems, and lack of sophisticated infrastructure in dealing with complex, market-driven financial arrangements. There is more to adequate access to health care than an insurance card, and public systems fill some important gaps. To investigate this issue the Foundation supported a study by Dr. Tracy Lieu of the users of public immunization clinics in Contra Costa County, California. Somewhat surprisingly to ail of us, she found that a majority of them had health insurance: 24 percent had private insurance and 34 percent had Medi-Cal.[3] (See Figure 3) Of those with private insurance, almost one third had at least partial coverage for vaccines, but still came to the public clinic—the site of "last resort." Indeed most families had sources of preventive care other than the clinic and would have preferred to receive their vaccines at these sources. They named a variety of barriers, including waiting times, cost (or their perception of cost—one of the features of the current health insurance market is that many people do not know what they are insured for), problems with transportation, and others.

4. Risk adjustment will be critical if our health insurance system is to serve the ill along with the healthy.

Although insurance underwriting reform will remove the most egregious examples of risk selection by insurers, it most assuredly will not remove their financial interest—indeed their financial imperative—to avoid enrolling people with chronic disease and seek healthy unless people with chronic disease bring with them sufficient resources to pay for their care. Imagine, if you will, a world after enactment of the underwriting reforms for which there seems to be general consensus: companies may no longer exclude individuals for preexisting conditions; community rating is mandated; insurance cannot be canceled because of the development or appearance of disease. These are ail reforms which I endorse and support. But how will such a system operate in the real world? Suppose Joe Jones has AIDS and has just been diagnosed with a condition known as CMV retinitis—an expensive and sight-threatening infection which will require life-long treatment. He would then be able to walk into the office of any local health insurer and demand that they issue him a policy. Furthermore, he could be assured that this policy will be at the community rate—say, $180 per month. All this, despite the fact that he, his physician, and the insurer all know that my care will require more than $180 per day for the next several! weeks. Now many insurer in his or her right mind would do everything possible not to develop specialized expertise in AIDS lest they acquire a reputation for this expertise and therefore attract more patients with AIDS, each one of whom will cost them substantial amounts of money. (See Figure 4)

If I have a case of "brittle" diabetes, or you are a severe asthmatic, what are the incentives for a health plan to develop new and innovative programs for our care? If a plan recruits doctors with such expertise and develops a program of excellence in care we (and our expenses) will flock to such plans and no extra money will flock with us. This conundrum—how to collect money from individuals (perhaps via their employers) equally, yet pay it out to providers in accordance with differing need is at the heart of the fears of patients and providers alike about the system as it is now developing. Capitated arrangements with prepaid care may work fine for those health conditions which may arise at random and unpredictably—say, brain tumors, or are relatively minor cost, like a broken arm. But if the poor, the old, and the sick are not to be assiduously avoided even by the most well-meaning of health plans, then the incentives to attract and retain them must be built into the system. This is why the development and implementation of some practical scheme of prospective risk adjustment and retrospective reinsurance must be one of the most urgent intellectual and operational tasks facing health policy makers in the next few years.

To summarize, I believe that the confluence of legislative Reform and market reform creates six priorities for a successful attack on the problems of the underserved:

1. The development, support, and evaluation of new models of managed care which can address the challenges of providing efficient, high quality health care to underserved urban and rural populations. Such models must come both from organizations specifically created to meet this need (some exciting examples of which you will hear about today) and from the adaptation and evolution of more mainstream organizations.

2. The continued development of objective standards of quality to which health plans can be held accountable. There is a great deal of promising activity in this area, such as the evolution of "report cards". But without government intervention there may be insufficient incentive in the private sector alone to promulgate standards in such areas as care of complex diseases such as HIV and in fields such as family planning, mental health, and substance abuse which are of particular concern to low-income populations and in which the public sector currently plays a major role.

3. The development of standards for judging the adequacy of so-called enabling services which are medically necessary, such as transportation, outreach, and translation. Some of these services are currently reimbursed by Medicaid and are vital to the delivery of high quality care to individuals such as those with disabilities.

4. Strengthening legal protections and avenues of expeditious appeal and redress for consumer/policyholders. I believe that the vast majority of managed care plans are honest, capable, and want to provide the best possible care for their members. But there are tremendous sums of money at stake in this industry, and we are all aware that some grievous abuses exist. Furthermore, even with the best of intentions the sheer size of the plans now in existence and in formation brings with it a certain amount of bureaucracy, and bureaucracy can breed inertia and red tape. Even sophisticated and well-educated people can be brought to their knees by such systems at times.

5. The protection of safety net institutions and categorical programs during this transitional period, and the provision of financial and technical assistance to aid their adaptation to the new market and reimbursement realities. I do not here advocate permanent "spotted owl" status for any current arrangement. Indeed, I think that it is inevitable that some institutions and programs will shrink or disappear altogether if insurance coverage is significantly expanded. I hope that the poor, the chronically ill, residents of inner-cities and rural areas will have their choice of a variety of providers and plans. I therefore do not believe that any existing provider—or class of providers—can or should be guaranteed survival in the brave new world which we are entering. But the traditional providers of the poor must be given an opportunity to compete successfully. These institutions have taken years and decades to develop; many of our country's most vulnerable populations are highly dependent upon them for care, and it is doubtful that private market mechanisms will ever be willing and able to meet their needs. It therefore would be foolish to disregard the future of these traditional providers of care to the underserved.

6. The institution of mechanisms for spreading risk and adiusting payments to plans and/or providers to reflect the level of illness of the patients for whom they are responsible. Time does not permit an extensive discussion of this complex and technical matter, and I am no expert. But by some rnechanism—purchasing alliances, risk pools—there are a number of approaches—this issue must be dealt with or without sweeping hearth care Reform. If not, we will continue down a path on which providers and plans who do what we want them to do—develop expertise and learn how to optimally manage care, not enrollment, will be increasingly penalized for doing so. Indeed, the prohibition of overt redlining in insurance will mean that

plans will be forced, by the logic of adverse selection, to find ever-more-subtle ways to meet to some populations and avoid marketing to others.

In conclusion, I commend the Senate Finance Committee for its attention to the issue of health care reform. I particularly thank you for convening this session to address the needs of people whose voices are not the loudest and whose political clout perhaps not the greatest.

Addressing the inequities in the current system and creating a balanced system of incentives and safeguards to protect the interests of the underserved will inevitably require the creation of new institutions and mechanisms which will have to be tested in practice. Such a task is always daunting, but there simply is no alternative, for the existing mechanisms—whether market or regulatory—are not sufficient to solve these problems. I urge you, therefore, to be bold as well as prudent. Innovation will, I know, bring sharp criticism and entreaties for caution, because the economic and political stakes are so high. 8ut innovation is what is needed. Niccolo Machiavelli, who knew a thing or two about politics, might have Health Care Reform in mind when he said:

". . . . there is no more delicate matter to take in hand, nor more dangerous to conduct, nor more doubtful in its success, than to set up as a leader in the introduction of changes. For he who innovates will have for his enemies all those who are well off under the existing order of things, and only lukewarm supporters in those who might be better off under the new. This lukewarm temper arises partly from the fear of adversaries who have the laws on their side, and partly from the incredulity of mankind, who will never admit the merit of anything new, until they have seen it proved by the event. The result, however, is that whenever the enemies of change make an attack, they do so with all the zeal of partisans, while the others defend themselves so feebly as to endanger both themselves and their cause."[4]

Thank you very much.

REFERENCES

1. CBO Memorandum. Effects of Managed Care: An Update. Congressional Budget Office. March, 1994.
2. Summary Findings: Survey of Americans of Low Income. Kaiser-Harvard-NORC Survey, February 1993.
3. Lieu TL, Smith MD, Newacheck PW, et al. Health insurance and preventive care sources of children at public immunization clinics. Pediatrics 93(3):373–378, 1994.
4. Machiavelli N. The Prince. Dover Publications, Inc., New York.

Sources for Figures:

Bransome Jr ED. Financing the care of diabetes mellitus in the U.S. Diabetes Care 15 Supplement(1):1–5, March, 1992.
Health care reform for Americans with severe mental illnesses. Report of the national Advisory Mental Health Council. American Journal of Psychiatry 150(10):1447–1465, 1993.
Hellinger FJ. The lifetime cost of treating a person with HIV. JAMA 270(4):474–478, 1993.

Summary Findings: Survey of Americans of Low Income. Kaiser-Harvard-NORC Survey, February 1993.

The 10 problems ranked most serious by Americans with household income less than $20,000

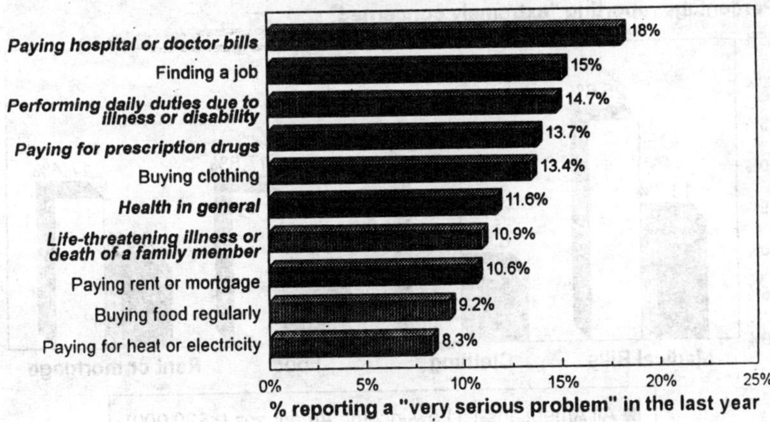

Source: NORC/Kaiser/Harvard Survey

Proportion of Americans who are extremely concerned about their ability to afford basic needs _in the next year_

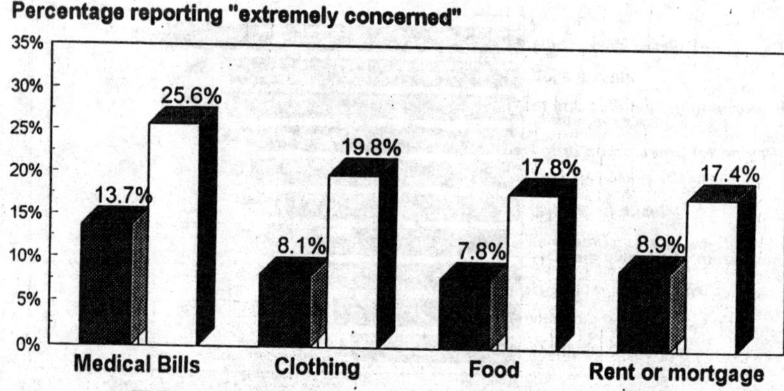

Source: NORC/Kaiser/Harvard Survey

Insurance Status of Public Immunization Clinic Users
Contra Costa County, CA
Fall, 1992

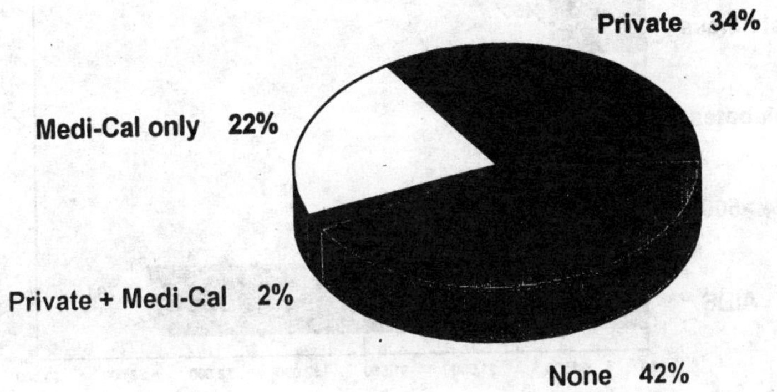

Source: Lieu, Smith, Newacheck. *et al*

Figure 4

Average Monthly
Health Care Costs

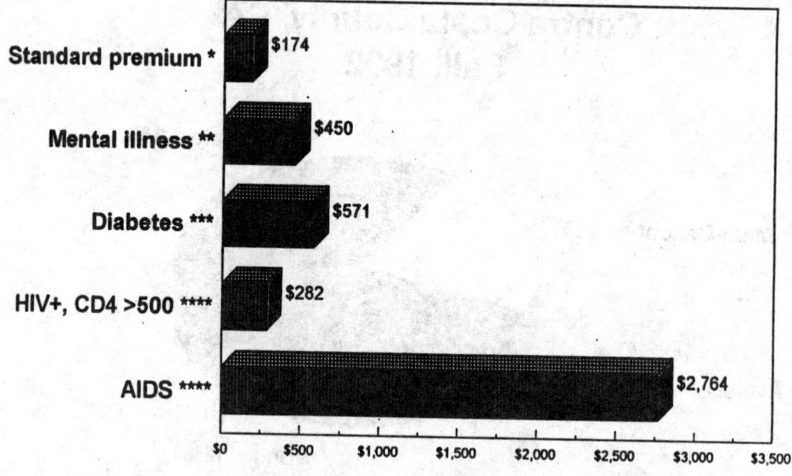

Sources: * FEHP (Ca..) '93/94 weighted avg.   *** Bransome
          ** Nat. Adv. Mental Health Council   **** Hellinger

RESPONSES OF DR. MARK D. SMITH TO A QUESTION FROM SENATOR PRYOR

Questions: In a recent report by the Association of Academic Health Centers, the author of a piece on urban health access problems indicates that we need what he calls "an urban practioner": someone schooled in primary care, in public health, and in the epidemiology of disease in the urban environment.

Would you agree with this author's assessment that we need specially trained provider to work. in an urban environment? Do we need a specially-trained provider to work in a rural environment?

Answer: I agree that patients in urban settings should expect that their providers be trained in both the epidemiology and psychosocial particularities of their diseases and their circumstances. So, too, should people in rural settings (and, for that matter, in suburban and other settings). I am, however, a bit skeptical about the capacity of undergraduate or even graduate professional education in such fields as medicine or nursing to adequately perform this task. Certainly there are ways in which these educational experiences can be improved to give students a better understanding of the environments in which they will be working, but many aspects of providers' practice are clearly molded more by their practice environments, continuing education (or lack thereof) and other influences, rather than the education they may have received years before. For this reason, it is particularly important that managed care organizations, which will increasingly dominate the practice environment and outlook of most practitioners in the next decade, be sensitive to these issues in their operations.

PREPARED STATEMENT OF EDWARD A. ULLMANN

Mr. Chairman, Members of the Committee, my name is Ed UIlmann, and I am President and CEO of WellCare, Inc., which has operated a successful Health Maintenance Organization (HMO) in rural upstate New York since 1983. I want to thank you for the opportunity to contribute WellCare's hard-won experience to your deliberations on health care.

WellCare, an IPA-model HMO (Individual Practice Association), currently has 75,000 members enrolled in the Hudson River Valley region from New York City to Albany and west into the Mohawk Valley and Leatherstocking Regions. WellCare offers health care services to a cross section of rural, suburban and small urban communities with a focus on small group enrollment and the enrollment of Medicaid recipients.

What makes WellCare special is that it works. WellCare has made a real difference for our members. I believe our successes and the lessons we have learned over the last decade can help point the way to making health reform work in rural America as a whole.

The problems associated with providing quality health care services in rural America are many and varied. They include: a shortage of primary care providers, professional isolation of providers from one another, the challenge of keeping health care affordable, management of technology, continuity of care, and lack of opportunities for continued training for providers.

WELLCARE'S MISSION

Early on WellCare established for its employers, providers, members, policymakers, regulators, shareholders, employees and community a very clear mission to guide all decision making. That mission is: to restructure the regional health care delivery system to make it work for our kids. Here is how WellCare has gone about achieving that mission.

THE VANISHING FAMILY DOCTOR

Restoring Primary Care in Rural America

For rural areas, the shortage of primary care providers—the vanishing family doctor—is a central problem. It is only through availability and regular access to HMO physicians that members can enjoy the preventive care and early diagnosis and treatment that both improves patient outcomes and controls health care costs. The primary care physician is the key member in the whole system of managed care.

Yet under the nation's current health care system, PCPs face a range of negative pressures including lower income than their specialist colleagues and life style issues resulting from the extreme demands on their time and energy. That is why less than a third of American physicians are in family practice, and why medical schools are still turning our more specialists than PCPs.

WellCare is both revitalizing and reinventing the old idea of the family doctor through strong support of current WellCare primary care practices, recruitment of new PCPs, and innovations in primary care.

Recruitment—Rural areas need more doctors. WellCare is the most aggressive recruiter of physicians in the region. In 1993, WellCare added 110 additional primary care physicians to its network and, over the past two years, has assisted 22 doctors to relocate to the Hudson River Valley.

Practice Support—As the dominant HMO in its area, WellCare is committed to reinvesting financial and human capital into our service area's whole structure of primary care with the goal of helping primary care physicians achieve success, control costs and provide high quality of care.

Through WellCare Medical Management, WellCare provides a wide range of support to current and start-up PCP practices depending on their individual needs. WellCare operates several primary care practices, administering all the day-to-day operations. In other cases, WellCare helps with facility renovations or capital expenditures for new medical equipment or provides consulting and marketing services. WellCare also is creative in the compensation packages it offers its PCPs to be better responsive to each particular PCP's family's financial needs.

WellCare helps equip and train its PCP practice to utilize computers to electronically transmit and receive encounter data, claims information, referral authorizations, orders for laboratory tests and more. This also streamlines service to members and facilitates our own data collection.

Professional Outreach—WellCare's Ambassador. Program brings on-site help in managed care to primary care practice staffs by means of roving ambassadors who crisscross the WellCare service area. WellCare Ambassadors assist the providers' staff in communicating policy and procedures to patients and also train the staff in the practices of managed care.

Professional and Community Education—WellCare Conferencing actively participates in the continuing education of physicians and mid-level providers, including advanced medical seminars with CME credits. There are also ongoing WellCare Health Forums and health education lectures for employers, members and the community-at-large, including updates on specialized topics such as breast cancer, diabetes and asthma control. These health care conferences are held throughout WellCare's service area and frequently in WellCare's own 120-seat lecture hall.

THE WELLCARE FAMILY HEALTH ALLIANCE

Organizing Primary Care in Rural America

While most HMOs compile lists of physicians, WellCare organizes them. One of WellCare's unique and innovative approaches to the needs of the primary care physicians and to members' health care is the formation of the WellCare Family Health Alliance, an organization of mutual support among primary care practices throughout the service area. Currently, the alliance includes sixteen practices serving some 80,000 patients about 28 percent of whom are WellCare members.

The WellCare Family Health Alliance provides:

* *Strong in-hospital coverage.* The Alliance includes designated, board certified in-hospital physicians who work closely with affiliated PCPs to provide in-patient coverage for their hospitalized WellCare members. This reduces the time a PCP has to spend at the hospital.
* *Improved member access to providers.* With PCPs relieved of hospital rounds, they are more accessible to patients at the office. Some Alliance practices have even been able to begin offering evening and weekend office hours.
* *Better on-call and emergency care coverage teams.* The formal arrangements for backup coverage among Alliance members means physicians work more efficiently together to dramatically reduce the strains on the PCP's family life of being accessible to patients 24 hours a day.
* *Integration of health care.* Health care does not begin and end with physicians. As the Alliance broadens to include specialists and even alternative providers such as acupuncturists, nutritionists, chiropractors, etc., WellCare will be able to provide members with a wide range of fully-integrated health services through Primary Care Teams headed by the PCP.
* *Cost control through global budgeting and group purchasing.* Cost containment can be enhanced through the economies of scale made possible by the Alliance.
* *Improved regional health planning.* The Alliance makes possible for the first time a regionwide mechanism for health care planning, creating enormous potential for improved preventive care and outcomes improvement.

- *Improved data collection and medical outcomes measurement.* The Alliance permits more comprehensive and consistent gathering of data, which can contribute to the overall managed care process. 4

CAPITATION AND RISK-SHARING

Controlling the Costs of Primary Care in Rural America

Capitation is an integral part of WellCare's approach to managed care both for cost containment and because of the way it helps reallocate health care resources to preventive medicine. Capitation is the single most important tool for making health care better and more affordable at the same time.

HMOs in the East commonly negotiate discounted fees to control costs, but WellCare is one of the few fully-capitated HMOs in the region. WellCare currently has capitation arrangements with more than 90 percent of the PCPs in its provider network.

Simply put, capitation makes the PCP a partner with WellCare in controlling health care utilization and cost and emphasizing preventive care.

Under capitation, each PCP is paid a fixed monthly fee for each member who uses that physician. From this allocation of capitation money, each PCP must cover all the costs for medical services used by his or her member pool. Surplus money at the end of the year reverts to the physician, but the physician is liable for cost overruns as well.

With WellCare's system of "full" capitation, the PCP must pay not only for his or her own services, but for the costs of specialists to whom the PCP makes referrals as well. This further increases the PCP's responsibility for controlling utilization of services.

Under the old fee-for-service system, there is no economic incentive for physicians to practice preventive medicine. Instead, physicians get paid more when patients utilize more medical services. Coupled with the trend to practice "defensive medicine," the fee-for-service system has led to a serious overutilization of medical services and has dramatically driven up the cost of health care.

This rising cost has in turn resulted in patients putting off going to the doctor until they are sicker and require more costly treatment. The overall net effect has been spiraling health care cost increases in our country in recent decades and poorer outcomes for patients.

Under WellCare's capitation arrangements, physicians have a financial incentive to keep patients healthy and avoid costly medical services. Through low copayments, WellCare encourages members to see their PCP more often for check-ups and preventive care. The end result is that better preventive care improves the level of health for all patients; medical outcomes are better for patients whose illnesses are caught and treated early, and health care costs are kept under control.

In addition, WellCare's Quality Assurance Department rigorously reviews physicians' documentation, medical outcomes and other quality measure to assure that sound medical procedures are followed. And WellCare also has a formal set of procedures to review member, employer or provider complaints. Physicians with poor quality records ultimately will be dropped from WellCare's list of PCPs.

Even the best PCP can't prevent every serious illness. To spread the risks more evenly, a portion of each PCP's capitation fees is pooled with other PCPs' fees to help pay for members who need extensive medical care. This also eliminates any tendency to withhold health services when they are needed the most.

The capitation fee is negotiated annually with each PCP or practice and can vary according to the characteristics of the PCP's member base, the geographic region, the physician's specialty, utilization patterns, quality of care, member satisfaction and other factors.

Approximately 10 percent is paid directly to the PCP for primary care services; 43 percent is allocated for payment to specialists and other providers to whom the PCP refers patients; 40 percent is included in the risk-sharing account to cover in-area and out-of-area hospital expenses and individual member medical expenses that total more than $2,500 per year; and 5 percent goes into a catastrophic account to cover deficiencies in the risk-sharing account. The balance is set aside for preventive health measures, such as AIDS screening and special vaccinations.

WellCare plans to bring specialists into the risk-sharing structure. However, WellCare currently negotiates favorable rates with specialists some 20 to 40 percent below usual and customary fees.

Our focus on individual capitated or risk-sharing contracts with primary care physicians resulted in a medical loss ratio at year end of 80.2 percent down from 81.6 percent for 1992. WellCare fostered a partnership of trust between provider and insurer that is seldom seen in managed care. Capitation efficiency was increased with the introduction of computerized claims submission (Claims Express) and telephone authorization for necessary medical referrals (Auth Express). As WellCare continues to increase its market share, especially in the Hudson River Valley, its ability to negotiate favorable provider contracts increases accordingly.

WELLCARE'S QUALITY ASSURANCE PROGRAM

The Cost-Quality Equation in Primary Care

Pervading all of WellCare's organizational structures is a clear focus on Quality as the ultimate measure of health care. The highest quality health care will keep members in better health through prevention, will result in better outcomes through early diagnosis and treatment, and ultimately will cost less.

WellCare's Quality efforts and our entire health care delivery program recently received Provisional Accreditation from the National Committee for Quality Assurance (NCQA).

HEALTHY CHOICE: MANAGED CARE FOR THE MEDICAID POPULATION

Quality, Low-Cost Primary Care for Entitlement Groups

The Healthy Choice program is WellCare's model program for providing high quality, cost-effective and dignified health care for Medicaid recipients. Healthy Choice has enrolled almost 9,000 Medicaid recipients into managed care, bringing medical care to many members of this underserved population for the first time. The program is growing at the rate of approximately 250 members per month.

Healthy Choice is an alternative form of health care delivery to the costly traditional Medicaid fee-for-service system and reliance on Emergency Room care. The program's implementation is a joint effort between federal, state and local governments, and compensation is provided to WellCare on a fixed monthly age/sex adjusted premium basis.

Healthy Choice provides a full range of hospital, medical, and prescription drug coverage to Medicaid enrollees, specifically Aid to Families with Dependent Children (ADC) recipients, Home Relief (HR), and Medicaid Only.

Each Healthy Choice member establishes a close relationship with a primary care physician (PCP) from our network of private practice physicians in the fields of family practice, internal medicine, and pediatrics. Through the PCP, the member has access to a wide range of specialty care on a referral basis.

The Healthy Choice program stresses the same philosophy of care as WellCare's other programs: access to continuity, appropriateness, and quality of care. Emphasis is placed on the management of preventive care, early diagnosis, treatment, and follow-up care. The program stresses minimizing the use of the emergency room and maximizing primary care services.

Healthy Choice encourages and monitors member care as related to the New York State Department of Health's Prenatal Care Standards, Child TeenHealth Plan, Family Planning Service, and Reproductive Health requirements.

Benefits of Healthy Choice are:

For Government—

* Budget predictability and cost containment through capitated agreements.
* Primary care entry into an integrated health care delivery system with built-in quality assurance programs for all Medicaid recipients.
* Cost savings in reduced claims processing costs, out-of-area transportation costs, and a savings over existing Medicaid fee-for-service costs. According to the New York State Department of Social Service's cost analysis (June 1993), there is an average cost savings of 14.30/0 for managed care enrollees, compared to fee-for-service Medicaid recipients.
* Increased accountability for customer satisfaction and effectiveness (in terms of impact on clinical status, function, and well-being) of medical services.

For Health Care Providers—

* Input into the decision making process.
* Removal of government as the middleman.
* Relief for hospital emergency rooms formerly burdened by Medicaid recipients.
* Access to medical outcomes and practice guidelines.

For Medicaid Recipients—

* Choice of a personal primary care physician with seven-day a week, 24-hour on-call coverage.
* Enhanced dignity with WellCare ID card and access to WellCare member benefits.
* Increased acceptance by physicians.

- Access to local medical specialists including a personal OB/GYN.
- High quality care, including preventive care.
- Access to a member service team that handles problems or concerns in a timely and dignified manner.
- Assistance in obtaining transportation for provider office visits, appointment scheduling, and dealing with language and cultural barriers.
- Access to case management and quality assurance departments that monitor care related to family planning and reproductive health, high-risk pregnancies, and coordination of medical treatment for conditions such as AIDS or cancer.
- Assistance with helping to integrate health care services with community social services related support resources. This assistance includes WIC referrals, school nurse programs, Child Teen Health requirements, Maternal-Infant Service, Planned Parenthood and Infant Health Program.

WellCare's Healthy Choice Program has demonstrated that Medicaid managed care does indeed increase access to high quality care for recipients and is not just government's way of pushing poor people into capitated delivery systems for cost containment and enhanced budget predictability

WellCare's Healthy Choice Medicaid managed care program is successful because it is the right thing to do.

RECOMMENDATIONS

WellCare believes that the challenges of health reform, especially in rural America, can be met if we can implement nationally some of the following ideas:

- First, nationally celebrate the primary care physician and the specialty of preventive medicine. Make expansion of primary care physicians the cornerstone of health care reform and encourage innovative ways to increase their economic compensation. This should include the establishment of a percentage of all savings realized by global budget arrangement to be returned directly to the primary care team.
- Encourage HMOs and related managed care organizations continue to develop models to improve the quality of life for primary care physicians, especially those in solo practice. WellCare's efforts to form regional health alliances have been extremely successful in achieving this goal, especially in the areas of increasing the amount of time available for ambulatory services, alleviating professional isolation, and to overall begin to make medicine fun again for the physician. Quality of life issues. rather than economic issues. are the number one way to retain and increase primary care providers in rural America. Quality of life issues gain importance as more and more women—with their own strong family bonds—join the ranks of providers.
- Establish one-year primary care residency programs to help retrain specialty care physicians in primary and preventive care.
- Change medical residency programs to become two-thirds inpatient training and one-third outpatient/managed care training. Expand use of qualified HMOs as residency training sites.
- Establish statewide primary care scholarship funds in partnership with the private sector.

Retire all medical student loans for a new physician in return for a five-year commitment to practice primary care in designated areas.

- Assist primary care physicians to be better decision makers through information systems, education, medical outcomes and strong quality assurance programs.
- Develop innovative models to provide independent primary care physicians financial protection through guaranteed minimum income employment agreements.
- Expand the training of mid-level providers, especially physician assistants, to assist primary care physicians with more than 50% of their functions at a lower cost.
- Build new models for primary care delivery in this country that would include a wide range of health professionals trained in alternative therapies working as a team under the direction of a primary care physician. In rural America, we cannot afford to isolate or exclude competent alternative primary care professionals from insurance participation simply because their training or philosophy may be outside the nationally recognized medical model. WellCare will soon be offering such therapies to our members in our Center for Wellness Program.

In conclusion, if our goal is to provide universal health care as a basic human right for all Americans, we can no longer tolerate our current fragmented and inefficient systems of care. We must immediately restructure our health care delivery systems around primary care and prevention, celebrating the innovative models for health care delivery that incorporate a focus on medical outcomes, quality assurance and accountability for cost containment.

In short, we must learn to work together, mounting a multidisciplinary team effort to create a health care system that recognizes that every patient is a full human being, not a collection of body parts.

Thank you for providing me the opportunity to present the WellCare story and our philosophy for restructuring the American health care delivery system in rural America. WellCare stands ready to help the Committee, the Congress and the Country in this important work.

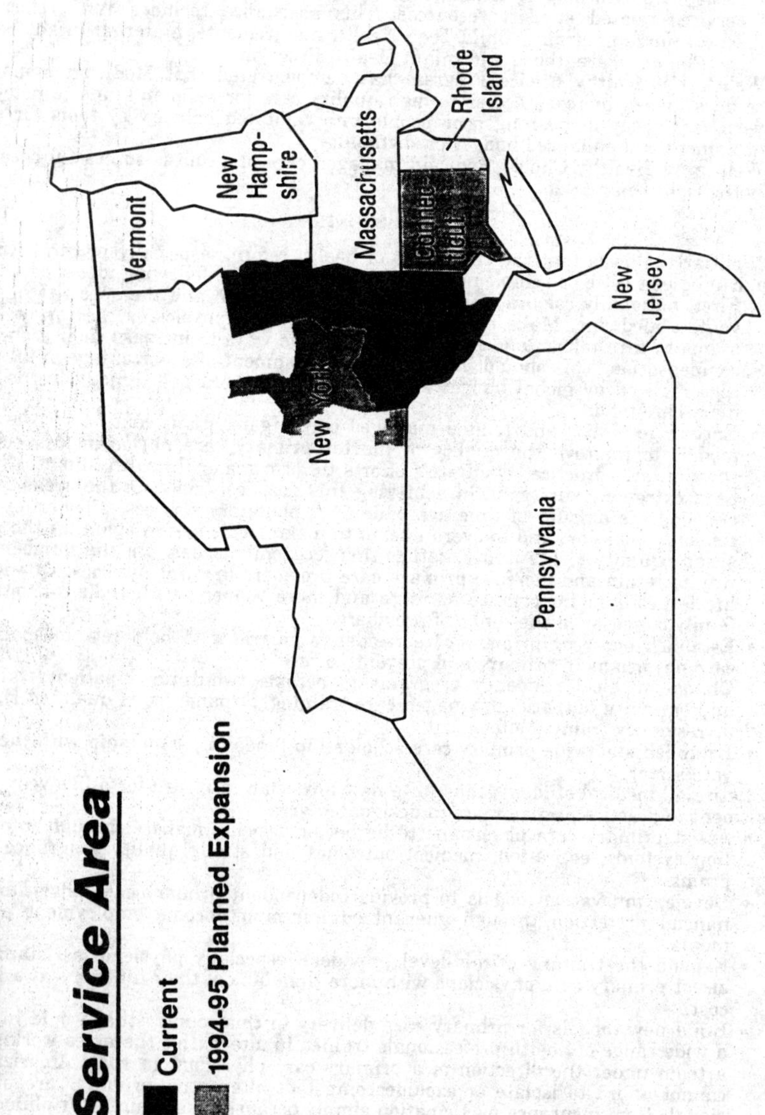

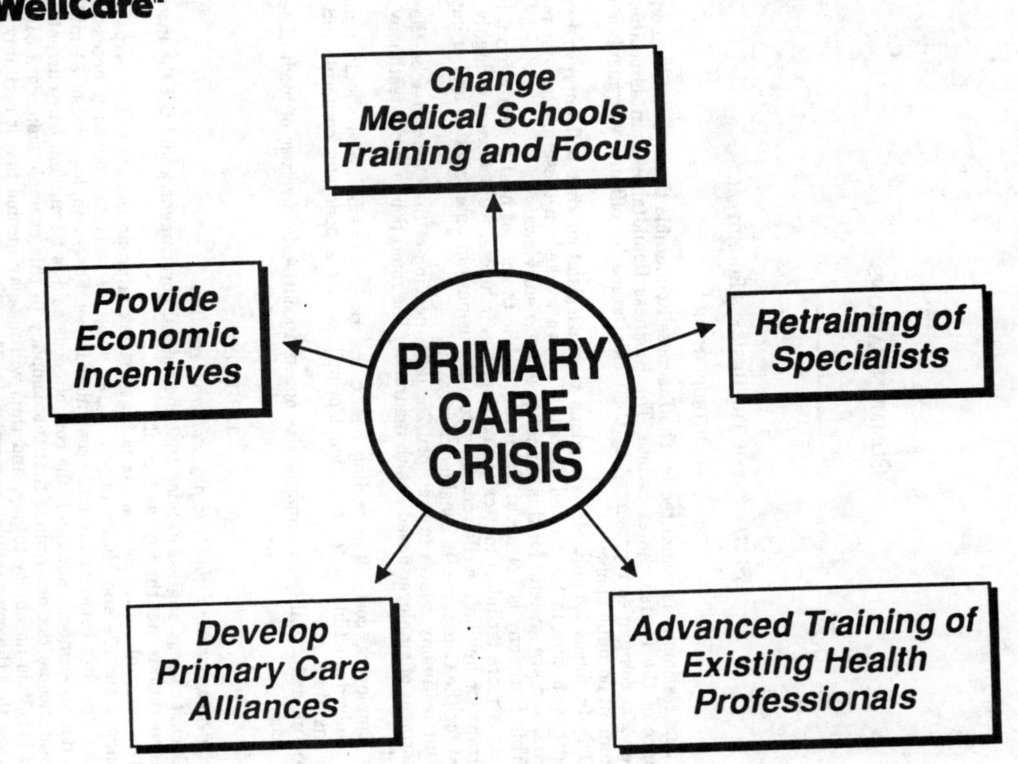
WellCare™
Change
Medical Schools
Training and Focus
Provide
Economic
Incentives
PRIMARY
CARE
CRISIS
Retraining of
Specialists
Develop
Primary Care
Alliances
Advanced Training of
Existing Health
Professionals

COMMUNICATIONS

STATEMENT OF THE BUSINESS ROUNDTABLE

INTRODUCTION

This testimony is submitted by The Business Roundtable to the Committee on Finance of the United States Senate. The Business Roundtable is an association of over 200 companies represented by their chief executive officers, who monitor and comment on public policy.

The Business Roundtable is anxious to see legislation that will improve health and health care in the United States. We have worked on these matters for many years, and are grateful for this chance to express our views.

This testimony is not about the broad, public themes of health care reform. It is about a more technical matter of taxation. Nevertheless, we believe it is highly important for having a well-ordered system of business income taxation and is important for the Committee to consider closely.

Our testimony relates to the April 26, 1994, hearing of the Committee on the tax treatment of employer-based health insurance. The main points of our testimony are that

- Employers' costs of providing health insurance for employees should remain fully deductible under traditional principles of tax policy for corporate income taxation, and
- Full deductibility by employers is not an incentive for overuse of medical services.

TESTIMONY

Income tax based on ability to pay, not gross receipts

Decades ago, Congress decided that the federal government would tax the income of corporations, not their gross receipts.

The rationale of an income tax is that the tax is proportionate to the taxpayer's economic success and ability to pay. A tax on gross receipts would not necessarily make this link between tax and economic success. For example, sales of $1 million are not an economic success if the cost of goods sold is $2 million. Our current corporate income tax determines that the company in this example suffered a $1 million loss, has no ability to pay, and thus will not pay income tax; it certainly does not say that the company will pay tax on its $1 million of receipts.

Deductions necessary for an income tax

The basic difference between a tax on business income and a tax on business receipts is that income is measured net of business expenses. The expenses are deductible in full. It is necessary for these expenses to be deductible in full as a matter of tax policy, if the policy objective is to tax business income.

Deductions for compensation of employees

Compensation of employees is a significant business expense. Some compensation is paid as directly wages, and some is paid as health benefits and other benefits for employees. However it is paid, the compensation of employees must be deducted from gross receipts in order to determine the income of employers, and it must be deducted in full.

Therefore, our testimony regarding the tax treatment of employer-based health insurance is for the uncompromised application of standard income tax policy and principles, which require the full deductibility of the employers' cost without caps, phase-outs, or other dilutions.

Is deductibility a subsidy or incentive?

Some who may not have the Committee's experience in taxation contend that the employer's deduction for health insurance payments is a "subsidy" or " incentive" to overuse health care. They say that if the federal government wants to contain inflation of health care prices, it should cap or limit the employer's deduction so that employers will be less willing to participate in more expensive plans.

Our response is that this line of thinking totally misconstrues the purpose of expense deductions in a business income tax, and that the Committee should be definite about rejecting it so long as Congress wishes to tax income for its primary stream of revenue.

Of course, deductibility is very important for an income taxpayer in the 35-percent bracket, because the loss of deductibility for a certain business item would raise the item's after-tax price to the taxpayer by over 50 percent. For example, automakers would see steel as costing them more and would use less of it, if Congress made their payments for steel nondeductible. But that observation does not mean that the tax system is subsidizing manufacturers to buy "too much" steel, and it certainly does not mean that limitations on the deductibility of payments for steel would be a sensible policy for reducing the use of steel.

We reiterate the main point: the full deduction of employer's costs of compensating employees is a necessary ingredient of a tax system that seeks to tax business income and ability to pay rather than gross receipts.

The deduction is not a subsidy or incentive to buy health care for employees instead of paying cash wages in the same amount, because employers currently take the same deduction for either type of compensation.

STATEMENT OF THE RURAL HEALTH NETWORK COALITION

The Rural Health Network Coalition (RHNC) is pleased to have the opportunity to submit testimony for the record of the Senate Finance Committee's April 21, 1994 hearing on "Access to Health Care in Rural and Inner-City Communities Under Health Care Reform."

The RHNC is a 501(c)(3) corporation [1] with seven hospital members that are designated as Rural Referral Centers (RRCs) under Medicare's prospective payment system. RRCs are larger rural hospitals that provide secondary and tertiary health care services to rural populations.[2] The RHNC members exemplify larger rural health care institutions striving to lead the evolution of rural health care delivery to managed care and guaranteed access for rural populations to community-based, quality providers. The efforts of these hospitals to launch the development of rural health managed care networks in their communities also is illustrative of the need for federal health reform policy to recognize that these types of initiatives in many rural communities are in their infancy. As such, different approaches must be studied and adequate flexibility provided so that rural communities can experiment to assess which approaches will be most appropriate for their local needs. Finally, the RHNC membership is a reminder that sophisticated secondary and tertiary care hospitals are located throughout rural America (256 hospitals currently are designated as RRCs), poised to be central players in rural health care network development.

BACKGROUND ON RHNC

The RHNC hospitals began meeting in 1991 with an original mission to devise a legislative alternative to the Essential Access Community Hospital (EACH) program established by the Omnibus Budget Reconciliation Act of 1989. In the view of these hospitals, the EACH program is not a viable provider networking approach for the rural areas in which they operate because it imposes stringent guidelines on bedsize and length of stay at rural primary care hospitals (RPCH). In addition, the EACH program fails to address managed care strategies for rural communities. The RHNC members firmly believe that managed care should be pursued in rural areas as a mechanism for improving access and appropriate utilization of health care services for rural populations.

As the largest providers in their communities, and as entities with a pivotal role in the continued viability of rural America, the RHNC hospitals set forth to develop

---

[1] Application pending.

[2] The criteria for RRC designation include (i) 275 beds, or (ii) satisfaction of case-mix, discharge, and other medical staff, source of inpatients, or volume of referrals criteria. 42 C.F.R. §412.96.

a proposal for provider networking in rural America and for the integration of the financing and delivery of health care on a managed care basis. The hospitals met on multiple occasions, including with representatives from Capitol Hill, officials from the Health Care Financing Administration (HCFA), Office of Rural Health Policy, and representatives from the National Rural Health Association and the Robert Wood Johnson Foundation.

The hospitals determined that an acute need existed for proposals on rural health care delivery, especially in the context of health care reform where policymakers already were struggling to devise a health reform plan that could address the special needs of rural America. As providers with a strong financial base and critical mass to initiate provider networking and managed care, these RRCs perceived a responsibility as well as an opportunity to develop a provider networking proposal appropriate to rural America. In addition, these hospitals perceived a need to develop strategies for the incorporation of Medicare, and possibly Medicaid, beneficiaries into rural provider networks since these populations comprise a large percentage of most rural hospitals' patient base. The hospitals recognized that it would be prudent to pursue development of provider networks in the non-Medicare sector before pursuing a Medicare demonstration project so that non-RRC rural providers would become involved network participants and so that a foundation would be in place for the fold-in of Medicare beneficiaries.

By January of 1994, six of the RHNC members had completed feasibility studies and determined that development of provider networks intended to provide coordinated care to patients could be viable in their communities. These six members have submitted a formal proposal for a demonstration project in Medicare managed care to HCFA.[3] Network development activities differ in each location and members continue to exchange ideas and experience. The demonstration would present HCFA with the opportunity to study provider networking and managed care in six different rural locations and to learn from data gathered from all sites.

The RHNC members collectively possess broad knowledge about rural health care and many years of experience in managing the leading health organizations in six rural locations. The RHNC members have invested their own staff and material resources and have invited input from a variety of experts in order to study the issues of rural health care from both a practical and a theoretical perspective. With the submission of the demonstration proposal, the RHNC indicates its desire to put into practice and to evaluate several progressive initiatives designed to introduce managed care to rural areas, as well as to experiment with risk management. The diversity of the RHNC members brings depth to the project.

SUMMARY OF PENDING MEDICARE DEMONSTRATION PROJECT PROPOSAL

A rural managed care demonstration would be established in six sites in four states, designed to promote better access to health care for Medicare beneficiaries and to contain costs by establishing new Medicare payment structures for risk-sharing with participating providers. The demonstration would be parceled into three phases over four and a half years. Phase I (12 months) would be used to finish building provider networks, enroll Medicare beneficiaries, and generate options for new Medicare risk-sharing payment structures. During Phase II (18 months) all covered services would be provided to enrolled beneficiaries while operating under traditional Medicare payment rules. Medicare risk-sharing payment structures to be implemented in Phase III (24 months) would be negotiated with HCFA on a per site basis. The networks in each site would be entities formed or sponsored by or including non-profit RRCs. (These networks will be referred to as the "Provider Networks" and the RRCs will be referred to as "Sponsoring Entities.") The Sponsoring Entities would initiate the development of the Provider Networks that would form the foundation of the new managed care delivery systems in their areas under the demonstration. By the beginning of Phase III, an entity at each site would have become qualified under state law to accept risk and would meet all additional Medicare requirements for risk contracting (the "Risk-Bearing Entity"). This entity would integrate financing and delivery of health care for its enrollees.

Currently under development in each of the six sites, the Provider Networks would be established and maintained in all three phases of the demonstration and would provide, either directly or through arrangements with other providers, all Medicare covered services in Phases II and III of the demonstration.

A new Medicare Community Data System (MCDS) would be established for the project to develop outcome measures and provide feedback data on the basis of small

---

[3] Proposal submitted March 24, 1994 in response to HCFA grant solicitation published in the January 13, 1994 *Federal Register.*

area analysis. Patient level data from Medicare claims would be combined with health status, health risk, and other primary data gathered by plans or by survey. In Phases I and II, this data would be used by the Sponsoring Entities and HCFA to negotiate and establish new Medicare payment structures and to begin to study utilization and cost data. In Phase III, this data along with the data systems of the provider networks would be used by the Risk-Bearing Entities to monitor and profile provider utilization and outcomes and to credential participating providers. In many ways, the demonstration would be a "laboratory" for studying risk issues pertaining to health care delivery in rural areas; these risk issues include enrollment penetration, controllability of practice patterns, and risk-sharing between Medicare and Risk-Bearing Entities as well as risk-sharing between Risk-Bearing Entities and their participating providers.

The RHNC would coordinate the project and centrally would construct an outcomes management data system that would be used to provide Sponsoring Entities in Phase II and the Risk-Bearing Entities in Phase III with feedback on outcomes on a comparative basis. The Provider Networks would vary in structure and operation, though each would be organized to provide controlled access to secondary services and to provide improved access to primary services in the more thinly populated regions served. The RHNC also would coordinate the development of a standardized form to be utilized at all sites through which basic health care information would be gathered on each Medicare beneficiary at the time of enrollment and at annual anniversaries. The basic data would be used by the Provider Network and ultimately by the Risk-Bearing Entity and by HCFA to monitor health status and health risk.

Medicare beneficiaries voluntarily would elect to participate in the demonstration. Sponsoring Entities would recruit Medicare beneficiaries and providers. On a per site basis, beneficiaries would be offered enrollment incentives, such as claims assistance, vision and/or hearing testing and transportation. As incentives to participate in the Provider Network, providers would be offered assistance in attracting patients, billing, making referrals, receiving respite, and quality improvement assistance. All covered Medicare services would begin to be provided through the Provider Network in Phase II. At this stage, the Medicare beneficiary would choose a primary care physician who also would serve as the beneficiary's case manager. However, the beneficiary would not be penalized if he or she seeks care through providers other than the primary care provider until Phase III, the Risk-Bearing Phase.

During Phase II, providers who are participating in the Provider Networks would be reimbursed directly by Medicare under traditional Medicare payment rules. Based on data gathered during Phase II, the Sponsoring Entities would negotiate with HCFA risk-sharing methodologies and payment rates on a per site basis to become applicable in Phase III. In Phase III, the Risk-Bearing Entities would receive all Medicare payments for covered services rendered within the Provider Network according to the methodology and payment rates negotiated for each site. In Phase III, the program would work like other risk programs where Medicare services are covered only if provided through the Provider Network (other than emergencies or pre-approved referrals out-of-area). Medicare deductibles would be waived and copayments for primary care services modified in Phase III.

OTHER RHNC ACTIVITIES

The RHNC also is pursuing grants from several private foundations to facilitate network formation and the development of data information systems.

RHNC HEALTH REFORM PROPOSALS

1. Health reform should promote the development of health care networks and managed care in rural areas.

Due to the present under development of networks in many areas of rural America, it will be critical for health reform legislation to promote this development, through direct grants and demonstration projects. Testimony presented by CoreSource, Inc. to this Committee demonstrates that networking is possible in rural communities. The RHNC concurs with CoreSource's statement that the key to successful health care reform in rural areas is community-based, localized networks that limit referrals to out-of-area specialists and hospitals.

In order to accomplish this end, health reform legislation must provide financial support for the development of rural-based networks. The President's bill (H.R. 3600, S. 1757) envisions a Public Health Service initiative to develop plans and networks in medically underserved or health professional shortage areas. While this is a laudable proposal, it fails to recognize that even rural areas that are not designated as medically underserved or health professional shortage areas may need resource support to assist in the development of networks, especially managed care networks. Indeed, without the infusion of such resources, some rural areas may evolve into medically underserved or health professional shortage areas.

Senator Chafee's health reform proposal (S. 1770) would provide for demonstration projects to encourage the development and operation of rural health networks under the Medicare and Medicaid programs. The RHNC supports this type of initiative. However, the Chafee plan requires that private sector networks already be in place as a condition precedent for the conduct of a demonstration project. Since many rural areas are underdeveloped in network formation, they will need upfront assistance in developing networks into which Medicare and Medicaid populations can be folded. The RHNC members have recognized this reality and are in the process of network formation. However, multiple other rural areas have not taken this first step and may not do so without adequate encouragement and direct support from the government.

Another concern that must be addressed in health reform is the current inadequate Medicare managed care payment methodology (i.e., the average area per capita cost (AAPCC)). The RHNC members are concerned that this payment methodology, which is based on historic data, would so vastly underpay rural-based managed care entities for services that they would be nonviable. Senator Durenberger's bill, S. 1996, would provide for the development of a new Medicare managed care payment methodology. The RHNC supports this concept. However, the RHNC believes that, in rural areas, a variety of payment methodologies and different degrees of assumption of financial risk may be appropriate, such as would be explored through the RHNC's proposed demonstration. The RHNC also was pleased to see a provision in S. 1996 for health plans to receive an increased per capita rate for enrollees who reside in underserved rural areas.

2. Health reform expressly should recognize RRCs

None of the pending health reform plans expressly recognize the RRC designation nor the pivotal role that these hospitals must play in forging networks in rural America. Such recognition could be made in legislation regarding network formation in rural America. For instance, in the EACH legislation, RRCs are mentioned as hospitals which must be located at least 35 miles from an EACH, thereby recognizing that EACHs and RRCs may provide a similar breadth of services.

The President's bill would promote incentives for urban health plans to expand to rural areas. This approach is not the answer for rural communities. Rural providers, who are stakeholders in their communities, who understand local politics and needs, and who must live in rural communities, should be the leaders in rural health care delivery. Indeed, many urban institutions are struggling to adequately serve urban populations. They are unfamiliar with and uninvested in rural issues.

As evidenced by the RHNC's existence, rural providers, including RRCs, stand poised to become leaders in network formation in rural areas. Health reform legislation would be remiss in not recognizing this reality. The "essential community provider" designation, as conceived in the Clinton plan, would require health plans to contract with certain providers that serve low-income populations. At a minimum, RRCs which qualify as Medicare disproportionate share hospitals should be included among those providers who would qualify for this designation. Moreover, if the concept of the "essential community provider" is expanded to include providers other than those who serve low-income populations, RRCs should be among the providers categorized as "essential" and with which health plans must contract. Indeed, RRCs are essential providers to their communities for the provision of a wide range of health care services that rural populations otherwise would have to travel to urban areas in order to receive.

CONCLUSION

Health reform must promote reliance on community-based networks that localize care in rural America. In addition, rural areas need an infusion of financial resources to assist with network formation and to ensure that payment rates are sufficient to retain essential providers, including specialty providers such as RRCs, and to recruit and retain physicians. Finally, health reform expressly should recognize RRCs and their pivotal role in accomplishing the goal of minimizing the need to refer rural populations to urban areas for specialty care.

For further information, please feel free to contact the RHNC's Washington counsel, Sally A. Rosenberg or Wendy L. Krasner, at 202/887–8000.

SUBMITTED BY THE RURAL HEALTH NETWORK COALITION

MERLE WEST CORPORATIONS, Klamath Falls, Oregon David R. Arnold, CEO

REGIONAL WEST MEDICAL CENTER, Scottsbluff, Nebraska David M. Nitschke, President

GOOD SAMARITAN HOSPITAL, Kearney, Nebraska William W. Hendrickson, President/CEO

ST. FRANCIS MEDICAL CENTER, Grand Island, Nebraska Carl P. Bowman, Vice President, Fiscal Services

MEMORIAL HOSPITAL OF CARBONDALE, Carbondale, Illinois Jerry A. Hickam, Senior Vice President, CFO, Treasurer

NORTHERN MICHIGAN HOSPITAL, Petoskey, Michigan Jeffrey T. Wendling, President

ST. MARY'S HOSPITAL & MEDICAL CENTER, Grand Junction, Colorado Laurie Fehlberg, Director of Finance

---

STATEMENT OF THE RURAL REFERRAL CENTER COALITION

The Rural Referral Center Coalition (the Coalition) is pleased to have the opportunity to testify on the record of the Senate Finance Committee's April 21, 1994 hearing on "Access to Health Care in Rural and Inner-City Communities Under Health Care Reform." This informal coalition, which has been active in the federal arena for over nine years, represents the interests of hospitals designated as rural referral centers (RRCs) under the Medicare prospective payment system (PPS). Two hundred fifty-six hospitals currently are designated as RRCs and receive special payment adjustments under the Medicare PPS program in recognition of their additional costs in providing secondary and tertiary care to rural populations.[1]

The Coalition strongly believes that health reform legislation expressly should recognize RRCs as central players in health care delivery in rural America and as potential leaders in network formation in rural areas. Pending health reform proposals focus on the smaller providers in rural communities, such as rural health clinics, on the recruitment of physician and non-physician personnel to rural areas, and on medically underserved or health professional shortage areas. While these undoubtedly are key elements to the infrastructure of rural areas, so to are the providers, such as RRCs, that are positioned to forge rural-based networks. Indeed, RRCs are the rural health care providers that, by definition, provide local access to rural populations to a wide range of health care services, and, in so doing, localize care, minimize the need for referrals and travel to urban areas, provide services at costs lower than would be incurred in urban areas, and maintain rural economies because, without health care availability, the economies of many rural areas would flounder. In failing to recognize RRCs and to provide legislative support for their development of rural-based networks, pending health reform proposals risk jeopardizing not only these institutions which are the hubs for rural health care delivery in their areas, but also other rural hospitals and providers.

ISSUES AFFECTING RRCS THAT MUST BE ADDRESSED UNDER HEALTH REFORM

1. Universal coverage is not necessarily universal access

The Coalition supports guaranteed universal health insurance coverage for all Americans. We are concerned, however, that universal coverage is meaningless in rural America unless providers are geographically accessible to rural populations. As providers of primary, secondary and tertiary care in rural America, RRCs assure geographic access to residents of their immediate and surrounding rural communities. For instance, at Good Samaritan Hospital in Kearney, Nebraska, a 277 bed not-for-profit RRC, 58% of the admissions are patients who reside in rural areas outside of Buffalo County where the Hospital is located. The next closest hospital, which is 24 miles away, has an average daily census of three or less. If a broad range of services were not available at the Hospital, patients who use the Hospital's specialty services, including obstetrics, cardiology (open heart surgery), radiation therapy, nephrology, orthopaedics, gastroenterology, psychiatry and rehabilitation would have to travel an additional 130–200 miles to receive comparable care. The Hospital's primary and secondary service areas span 16 counties over 14,000 square miles, an area equivalent to the combined areas of Massachusetts, Rhode Island and Connecticut. The Hospital's full service area spans 44 counties, 17 of which do not have any hospitals and 13 of which do not have any physicians.

---

[1] The criteria for RRC designation include (i) 275 beds, or (ii) satisfaction of case-mix, discharge, and other medical staff, source of inpatients, or volume of referrals criteria. 42 C.F.R. § 412.96.

Indeed, RRCs offer both quality and cost-effective care for rural populations who otherwise would have to travel long distances for similar medical care. In some cases, this distance could mean the difference between life and death. In addition, the geographic accessibility of RRCs offers the intangible benefit of proximity to family members and saves families from costly stays in far away urban areas. Many rural residents elect care at RRCs over an urban hospital because they find rural providers to offer a more nurturing environment and cultural affinity.

A critical problem that has been identified in rural health care delivery is the dearth of physicians and non-physician professionals who are willing to locate in rural communities. Because RRCs are the larger rural health care institutions and offer a wide range of services, RRCs have proven ability in recruiting and retaining physician and non-physician professionals. In addition, RRCs are positioned to support and/or place primary care providers in outlying areas and spearhead network development and referral arrangements. For instance, East Alabama Medical Center, a 324 bed acute care not-for-profit RRC in Opelika, Alabama, has placed the only primary care physician in an outlying rural community with a population of 15,000. The community actually is closer to the Columbus, Georgia metropolitan statistical area than to East Alabama, but the Columbus hospitals have not taken any action to place a primary care physician in the community because of their assumption that the rural patients would travel to Columbus. East Alabama also has established eight cardiology outreach clinics in underserved rural areas within a 30 mile area, providing preventive and specialty services. Good Samaritan Hospital in Kearney, Nebraska has established four rural community clinics located from 20–70 miles from the Hospital, three of which are designated as rural health clinics. In one of these communities, the Hospital established the rural health clinic after the only local hospital closed down.

The Prospective Payment Assessment Commission (ProPAC) recently completed an informal study of the function of RRCs in their community. This study confirms that the RRC designation remains valid since these hospitals serve a critical role as providers of specialty care and services to vulnerable populations in rural areas. Attached is a series of charts prepared by ProPAC staff that elaborate on the role of all currently designated RRCs in their communities.

2. Rural America is not urban America

While there is widespread agreement that rural America has unique characteristics that demand special consideration under health reform, pending proposals do not adequately address these circumstances. For instance, those proposals which envision a competitive marketplace do not address the widely-acknowledged reality that most rural areas cannot support multiple health plans. Many rural areas do not have hospitals or physicians. In addition, rural populations tend to be comprised of a high percentage of Medicare (and Medicaid) beneficiaries, challenging the premise of pending health reform proposals that Medicare should remain a separate program, at least in rural America. Managed care entities are reluctant to accept risk contracts in many rural areas because, without Medicare beneficiaries, the enrollable population is too small to support a risk contract. Indeed, while managed care has become a significant presence in urban areas, it is barely a presence in most rural areas.

3. Rural providers should take the lead in rural health care delivery; a variety of demonstration projects in rural-based networks must be pursued before final legislation is adopted for rural health care

The President's plan would promote incentives for urban health plans to expand to rural areas. Historically, this approach has not worked for rural America nor is it the answer for the future of health care delivery in rural communities. Rural providers, who are stakeholders in their communities, who understand local politics and needs, and who must live in rural communities, should be the leaders in rural health care delivery. Further, if purchasing alliances or cooperatives are formed under health care reform, consideration should be given to forming separate alliances for rural populations to help ensure that the networks that serve these populations are rural, and not urban, based.

None of the pending proposals adequately would support the development of rural-based networks, including managed care networks. Financial support is needed to facilitate the development of networks in all rural areas. The President's bill would support the development of plans and networks in health professional shortage and medically underserved areas. However, this represents only a subset of rural America.

Senator Chafee's health reform proposal, S. 1770, would provide for rural demonstration projects to fold Medicare and Medicaid beneficiaries into existing rural-based networks. While such demonstrations are clearly needed, without support for the initial formation of these networks, it may not be feasible to establish these arrangements.

In addition, the current Medicare managed care payment structure, the average area per capita cost (AAPCC), needs to be revamped. This methodology inadequately reimburses managed care entities serving rural communities, which results in underpayments to rural providers serving Medicare beneficiaries in managed care plans. Senator Durenberger's proposal, S. 1966, would provide for a recalculation of the AAPCC, which the Coalition would support in concept. S. 1996 also would provide for a bonus in the per capita rate with respect to each enrollee who resides in an "underserved rural area," which is undefined.

In short, pending proposals should be combined and strengthened to provide financial support for the development of rural-based networks, in both the private and public sectors, and to study a variety of payment methodologies and risk-bearing strategies that may be appropriate for different rural communities. A series of demonstration projects should be pursued before any final legislative measures are enacted in rural health care delivery reform.

4. Medicare and Medicaid may need to be folded into health reform in rural America

As noted above, because Medicare and Medicaid beneficiaries comprise such a high percentage of the rural patient base, these programs may eventually need to be folded into reform in rural communities. For instance, at Northern Michigan Hospital, an RRC in Petoskey, Michigan, Medicare inpatient revenue represents 55% of total revenues. If the Medicare population cannot be folded in with private sector care, managed care entities will resist accepting risk contracts in areas such as Petoskey. Including Medicare and Medicaid beneficiaries in networks that serve the private sector also would ensure that hospitals would operate under the same incentives under both public and private programs.

5. Special payment adjustments may be appropriate for RRCs and other rural providers under health reform; further reductions in Medicare payments must be kept to a minimum

From the outset of Medicare PPS; Congress recognized that RRCs were critical to access to care in rural America. In 1993, Congress reaffirmed this by extending the RRC grandfather through hospitals' cost reporting periods beginning in federal fiscal year 1994. Medicare's special payment adjustments to RRCs were designed to ensure their continued role in providing geographic accessibility to a wide range of services for rural populations. Even with the upcoming elimination of the standardized amount differential, RRC status still has meaning and benefit under the Medicare program. Specifically, RRCs are eligible for special access rules under the Medicare Geographic Classification Review Board (MGCRB) and receive higher DSH adjustments than do other rural hospitals. Congress must maintain the RRC designation and the Medicare RRC payment adjustments and benefits that remain important to many RRCs.

Indeed, special payment adjustments may need to be devised for rural providers under health reform, including for RRCs, to ensure that rural populations have geographic accessibility to, not only primary care providers, but also specialty care providers which typically are essential to the economic viability of their rural communities.

At a minimum, there must be no further reductions in Medicare payments to rural providers. The American Hospital Association's recently released win-VHI study illustrates the potential impact on hospitals' operating margins of the Medicare reductions proposed in the President's plan. By the year 2000, the impact on all hospitals could be −28.9%, and the impact on RRCs as a group −29.3%. These reductions are unsustainable. For instance, at Northern Michigan Hospital, the proposed Medicare reductions would result in a total depletion of the Hospital's overall surplus last year plus one and a half million dollars. This.degree of revenue loss would cripple the Hospital's ability to forge needed rural-based networks and to continue to provide local specialty care to rural populations.

6. RRCs should be expressly recognized in health reform legislation, perhaps as essential community providers

The President's plan would require health plans to contract with "essential community providers" (ECPs). As drafted, such providers would be those that serve low-income populations. At a minimum, RRCs that qualify as Medicare disproportionate share hospitals should be included as ECPs as conceived in the Clinton plan. To the extent that the concept of ECPs is expanded beyond low-income providers, all RRCs should be considered ECPs since they are essential to the health care delivery system and economies of their rural areas.

If the ECP designation is not expanded, RRCs otherwise should expressly be recognized in health reform legislation as potential central players in forging rural-based networks. By way of example, the Essential Access Community Hospital (EACH) legislation adopted in the Omnibus Budget Reconciliation Act of 1989 expressly recognizes RRCs as hospitals from which EACHs must be located at least 35 miles. This provision implies that RRCs and EACHs are likely to offer a similar range of services.

7. Certain financial assistance will be needed in rural America to prepare for health reform

Rural-based networks will need financial assistance to develop communication and emergency transportation linkages. For example, East Alabama presently owns and operates an emergency transport and county rescue system, at a loss of $250,000 per year after accounting for subsidies.

8. Antitrust laws need to be reexamined as applied to rural providers

Antitrust laws should be reexamined as applicable to rural communities to maximize cooperative relationships amidst limited resources. Many rural providers do not pursue mergers simply because the legal fees in obtaining antitrust representation are so prohibitive.

9. Rural providers need protection from unreasonable financial risk

Finally, rural providers must be protected from unreasonable financial risk in order to assure that they offer geographic accessibility to rural populations. The RRC Coalition is extremely concerned that global budgets, spending targets, fee schedules and the use of historical spending as the basis for these mechanisms could result in significant underpayments which ultimately would erode further the provider base in rural America. Fair financing must be assured under health care reform for all providers, but particular attention must be paid to designing fair financing appropriate to the rural environment, given public policy priorities of assuring geographic access to quality care in rural communities.

Lawmakers must be mindful that health care providers are a basic element of the rural economic infrastructure. Since RRCs are fundamental to this health care infrastructure, every effort must be made under health reform to assure RRCs' continued role as providers of a broad range and depth of health care services in rural communities.

Attachment.

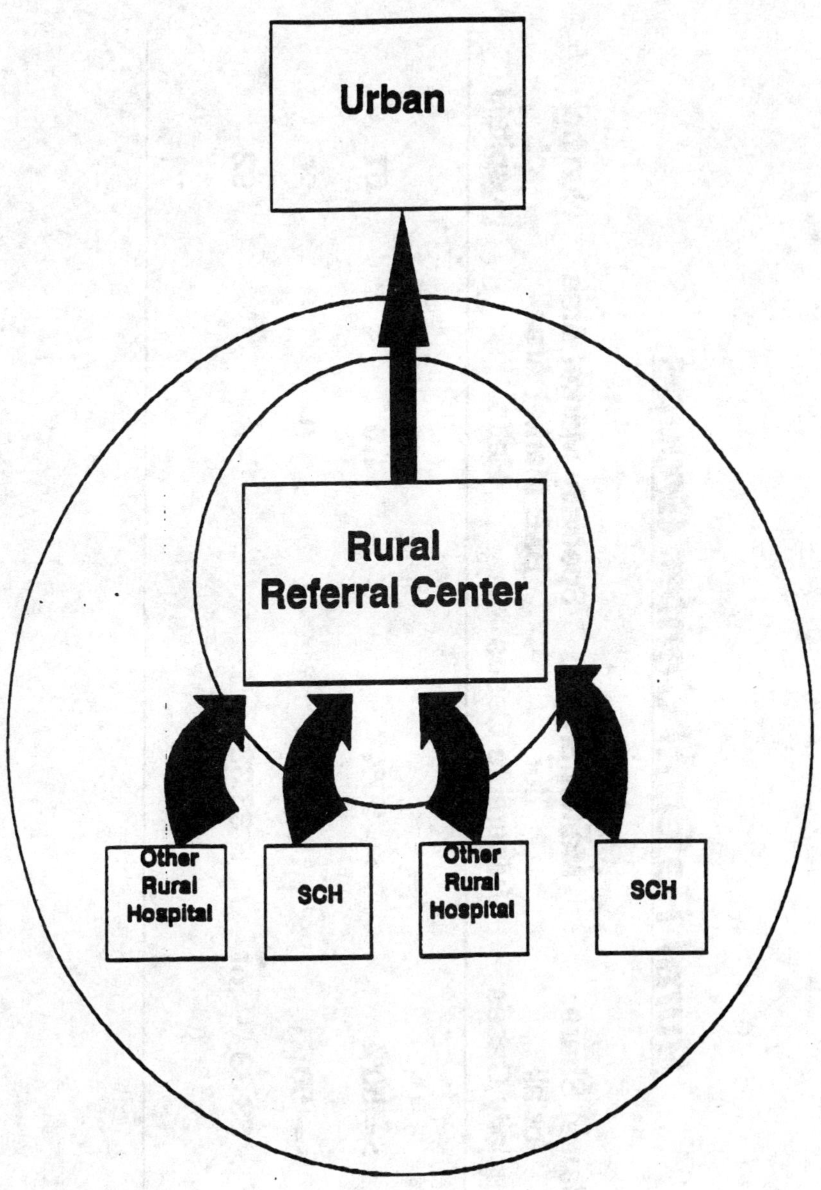

Urban
Rural
Referral Center
Other
Rural
Hospital
SCH
Other
Rural
Hospital
SCH

Rural Referral Center Groups

Group	Market Share for all Specialty Cases	Market Share for Vulnerable Cases	Specialty Market Area B&B Market Area Ratio	Number of Hospitals
A	>= 50%	>= 50%	>1.0	67
B (must have 2 out of 3)	>= 50	>= 50	> 1.0	26
C	> 33.33 or	> 33.33	-	92
D	-	-	-	71

Percent of Rural Referral Centers Providing Specialty Services

	A	B	C	D
CCU	27%	12%	26%	28%
ICU	99	92	97	99
Cardiac cath	39	38	45	61
Open heart surgery	9	4	14	25
Trauma	28	19	16	30
MRI	43	35	20	35
Radiation therapy	73	54	56	55
Outpatient surgery	99	96	100	100

County Characteristics of Rural Referral Centers

	A	B	C	D
Population density	101	106	93	102
Avg. Number of General Hospitals	1.6	2.8	1.8	2.2
Beds/1000 population	5.9	5.3	5.9	8.3
MDs/1000 population	1.5	1.3	1.5	2.3
Specialist/1000 population	0.4	0.3	0.4	0.7

Market Shares for Rural Rerral Centers

	A	B	C	D
"Bread and Butter"	77%	68%	56%	33%
Specialty Care	59	52	40	25
Vulnerable Cases	62	58	40	24

Specialty Market Area Characteristics

	A	B	C	D
Avg. number of other hospitals	1.1	1.7	3.2	6.1
Percent with:				
Teaching hospital	9%	12%	18%	31%
Other rural hospital	57	58	85	97
Another RRC	3	4	25	62
Avg. market area distance (in miles)	22.0	22.4	28.0	40.3
Avg. ratio of specialty market area to B&B market area	1.34	1.19	1.27	1.26

Financial Performance of Rural Referral Centers

	A	B	C	D
PPS margin	-6.03	-9.52	-1.69	-3.34
Total margin	5.45	6.04	6.34	6.93
Cost per case	$4374	$4509	$4231	$4766
Payment per case	4125	4117	4161	4612

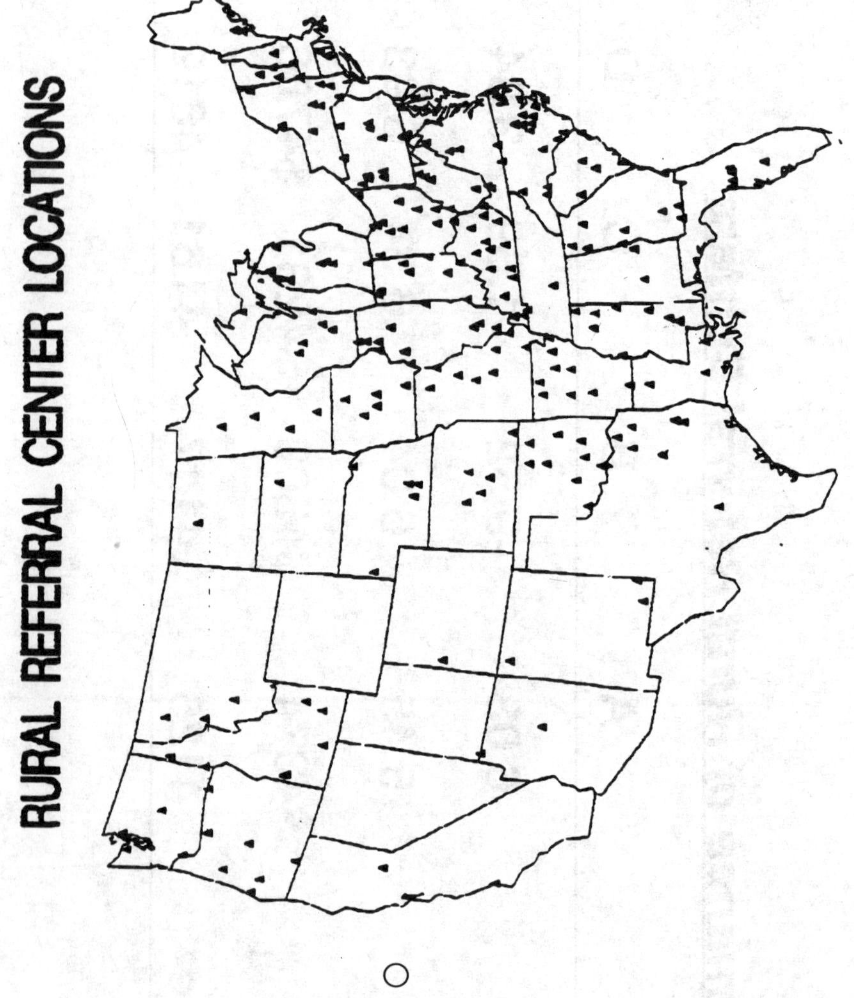
RURAL REFERRAL CENTER LOCATIONS

ISBN 0-16-048926-6
90000
9 780160 489266

APEX

TP_CF

76523826 -- 13